HIV&
SOCIAL
INTERACTION

HIV&
SOCIAL
INTERACTION

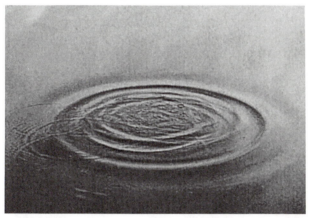

Valerian J. Derlega
Anita P. Barbee
Editors

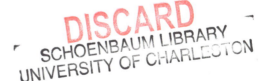

SAGE Publications
International Educational and Professional Publisher
Thousand Oaks   London   New Delhi

For information:

SAGE Publications, Inc.
2455 Teller Road
Thousand Oaks, California 91320
E-mail: order@sagepub.com

SAGE Publications Ltd.
6 Bonhill Street
London EC2A 4PU
United Kingdom

SAGE Publications India Pvt. Ltd.
M-32 Market
Greater Kailash I
New Delhi 110 048 India

Printed in the United States of America

Library of Congress Cataloging-in-Publication Data

Main entry under title:

HIV and social interaction / Valerian J. Derlega and Anita P. Barbee, editors.
    p. cm.
    Includes bibliographical references and index.
    ISBN 0-7619-0371-2 (cloth: acid-free paper)
    ISBN 0-7619-0372-0 (pbk.: acid-free paper)
    1. AIDS (Disease)—Social aspects. 2. HIV-positive persons.
  I. Derlega, Valerian J. II. Barbee, Anita P.
    RA644.A25 H5787 1988
    362.1′969792—dc21   98-8900

Acquiring Editor:	C. Terry Hendrix
Editorial Assistant:	Dale Mary Grenfell
Production Editor:	Wendy Westgate
Production Assistant:	Denise Santoyo
Book Designer/Typesetter:	Janelle LeMaster
Cover Designer:	Candice Harman

Contents

Preface

This book focuses on how the HIV infection affects the social interactions and relationships of the HIV-seropositive person. Our approach, which examines the social issues faced by the HIV-infected person in his or her daily life, complements other approaches that address the medical aspects of HIV and AIDS and the behavioral, psychological, and communication aspects of reducing "at-risk" behaviors that might transmit the HIV infection to others.

Although it is stressful enough to have a life-threatening disease like cancer or heart disease, individuals with the HIV infection also face social challenges based on other people's and society's reactions to the disease. For instance, many HIV-positive persons weigh carefully the decision about who, when, and how to tell someone about their seropositive status. Although disclosing HIV seropositivity to others may be associated with acceptance, caring, and social support from others, disclosing the HIV diagnosis may also lead to rejection and discrimination *by* others as well as emotional distress *for* others. The chapters in this book document—via the presentation of social interaction concepts and original research—how the HIV infection affects the seropositive person's relationships with family, friends, intimate partners, and others in his or her social network. Topics in various chapters include the stigmatization of HIV and AIDS; weighing the benefits and risks of self-disclosure about the HIV diagnosis; accessing, finding, and maintaining quality social support; the value of group residence facilities for persons with AIDS; the effects of HIV on intimate relationships; and the impact on volunteers of providing assistance to and having a close relationship with persons with AIDS.

We hope that the ideas and original research presented in this volume will be useful to a wide audience, including persons with the HIV infection, their friends, their families, their partners, and anyone who knows someone with HIV. The book should be particularly useful to students, social scientists, and health professionals who are interested in understanding and studying the social consequences of living with the HIV infection.

Some personal notes: This book has been in development for several years. The authors of the various chapters have shown considerable patience and perseverance in completing their chapters, and we the editors thank them for their participation.

During this time period, we have experienced both pain and joy in studying how HIV affects individuals' lives. Some people who were interviewed for the research reported in this book have died, and many were disabled by AIDS-related physical problems. On the other hand, the introduction of new drugs (including protease inhibitors) offers hope of extending the lives and the quality of life of many people with HIV infection, benefiting many individuals who participated in research described in this book's chapters. We owe a tremendous debt of gratitude to all the individuals who participated in the studies described in the book, and we dedicate the book to them.

Anita's motivation for working on this book and her sources of inspiration include two special people who graced her life for a time and who are now gone: Hugh Fleming, a high school classmate whose quiet, gentle, and graceful manner she always admired, and Mark Mims, a psychology graduate student at the University of Louisville whose sense of humor and laughter are emblazoned on her mind and heart forever. She would also like to dedicate this book to their memory.

We want to extend our thanks to the editorial staff at Sage Publications, including Terry Hendrix and Dale Mary Grenfell, for their support of this project. Finally we thank our partners, Barbara Winstead and Michael Cunningham, for supporting us during some of the stressful times that occurred while this book was being prepared.

—*Valerian J. Derlega*
—*Anita P. Barbee*

What Is the Impact of the HIV Infection on Individuals' Social Interactions and Relationships?

An Introduction

VALERIAN J. DERLEGA
Old Dominion University

ANITA P. BARBEE
University of Louisville

Let's go back approximately a decade in the United States. Consider the following illustration:

Ken found out that he had the human immunodeficiency virus (HIV) infection after his partner, Paul, was hospitalized and diagnosed with an acquired immune deficiency syndrome (AIDS)-related condition, *pneumocystis carinni* pneumonia (PCP). Paul, after struggling with a variety of illnesses associated with AIDS (the final stage of HIV, associated with severe immune deficiency), died a couple of years later. Ken, who found out about being HIV infected shortly after he contracted the disease, is still alive. He has been taking drugs to slow the spread of HIV in his body, as well as medications to fight off or prevent opportunistic infections and other medical conditions caused by advanced stages of HIV infection. At

1

the time this was written, Ken was in relatively good health: He benefited from enormous medical strides in the treatment of HIV, including
the development of medications to treat the opportunistic infections associated with advanced stages of HIV, the development of new antiretroviral therapies (including the combination of protease inhibitors in
"cocktails" with other antiretroviral drugs). These medical developments will, we hope, serve to improve the quality of physical life and
perhaps increase the prospects of long-term survival for Ken and many
others who are HIV infected.

Living with HIV has always meant coping with a progressive disease
that could eventually lead to death. Even now with new medical developments (Bartlett, 1996; Leland, 1996), living with HIV involves considerable uncertainty about the state of one's health. Whatever the physical health aspects of coping with HIV, HIV-infected persons have also
had to face challenges in their social relationships due to the disease.
These social aspects of coping with HIV are the subject matter of this
book.

The number of deaths due to AIDS has decreased recently among
those individuals using the antiretroviral combination therapies (Joyce,
1997). Nevertheless, the impact of AIDS has been enormous. For instance, by November 20, 1996, a total of 1,544,067 AIDS cases in adults
and children had been reported to the World Health Organization since
the beginning of this worldwide epidemic. Given the underreporting of
AIDS cases (e.g., individuals with AIDS may not recognize their own
health problems as AIDS related, they may be hesitant to tell others
about their health problems, or physicians may not report patients' AIDS
diagnoses to health authorities), it is estimated that there have been
about 8.4 million cases of AIDS worldwide from the late 1970s through
late 1996. Keeping in mind that HIV is the infection that causes AIDS,
and that many HIV-seropositive persons can live for many years without
any AIDS-defining clinical symptoms, there are about 22.6 million people who are living today with HIV or AIDS worldwide (World Health
Organization Global AIDS Statistics, 1997). Although it is difficult to
estimate the exact prevalence of HIV infection in the United States, there
may be anywhere from 600,000 to 900,000 people in the United States
living with HIV infection, most of them adults or adolescents (Centers
for Disease Control and Prevention [CDC], 1996a; Rosenberg, 1995;
see also Holmberg, 1996; Samuel & Osmond, 1996). Based on recent

statistics from the U.S. Centers for Disease Control and Prevention (CDC, 1996a), as of June 30, 1996, in the United States there was a cumulative total of 548,102 AIDS cases, and AIDS was one of the leading causes of death among persons aged 25-44 (CDC, 1996b). These approximate numbers of how many people are HIV-infected do not include the additional tens of millions of people worldwide who have known someone who is HIV seropositive or who have seen a family member, friend, partner, co-worker, or acquaintance die from AIDS (see, e.g., Geballe, Gruendel, & Andiman, 1995).

HIV infection and AIDS, like other life-threatening illnesses such as cancer and heart disease, exact a tremendous physical and psychological price on their victims and others who are in the victims' social network. Not only will the person with HIV, cancer, or heart disease have to worry about health complications and the possibility or inevitability of dying, there may be disruptions in relationships with family, friends, neighbors, people at work, or anyone the victim might meet. Living with HIV or AIDS, however, presents unique problems that are not normally experienced by someone who has cancer or heart disease. Reactions to someone with the HIV infection are influenced in part by cultural norms and stereotypes about behaviors associated with the transmission of HIV. For instance, in the United States, the most frequent routes of HIV transmission are (a) males having sex with other males and (b) intravenous drug use (CDC, 1996a), although worldwide, HIV is more likely to be transmitted via male-female sexual intercourse (American Association for World Health, 1996). Reactions to someone being HIV seropositive in the United States (and worldwide) are likely to be influenced by standards about the "cultural correctness" of various kinds of sexual behavior and attitudes about drug use (Pryor & Reeder, 1993; Shilts, 1987).

Let's return to our example of Ken to illustrate possible social consequences of living with HIV, especially in coping with others' possible disapproval and/or rejection.

Imagine that Ken works as a marketing executive for a large health insurance company. Ken has not told anyone at work about having the HIV infection. He thinks his knowledge about the HIV infection is a private matter, and the infection doesn't affect his work performance or pose any health risk to his coworkers. Ken does worry about the possibility that someone at work could possibly access his (or any employee's) health insurance records via the company computer and find out that he is infected (Davis, 1993). On the other hand, Ken has told a number of friends and associates about having the HIV infection, but he has decided not to tell some others. After Ken's partner, Paul, died, it took a year or more before Ken was willing to consider starting an intimate relationship. Ken met some individuals to whom he was sexually attracted, but he hesitated to start a relationship or even tell them about the HIV diagnosis for fear of their reactions to him when they found out. Ken decided on a "relationship strategy" based on *not* telling a possible relationship partner until he was certain that he wanted an intimate relationship with this person and was "sure" that this person wasn't likely to reject him. Ken also feels strongly that if he is going to have sex with someone, his partner will have to know about Ken's seropositivity and that they must use condoms.

Ken doesn't live in the same city as his parents or relatives, and it took him a couple of years before he told his relatives about his own HIV-positive diagnosis. Ken didn't tell his mom and dad about being HIV positive right away, partly because he might have to relive some of the difficulties he had when he disclosed to them that he was homosexual. Reactions of Ken's relatives to information about his HIV diagnosis have been mixed. Although many relatives expressed concern (including, in his mother's case, keeping informed about medical developments in the treatment of HIV and AIDS), at least one uncle reacted negatively, telling Ken's mother that Ken's lifestyle brought on the infection. This uncle has become less judgmental over time, but there is a mixture of worry for Ken's health, combined with unspoken tension among certain relatives, in the family's reactions to Ken's being HIV-infected.

A significant source of support for Ken has come from an HIV/AIDS support group sponsored by a local HIV/AIDS community service organization. Ken has developed strong friendships and loyalties with other members of the group—men *and* women who are also HIV positive. The group's meetings focus on a range of topics, from life insurance, medical developments and health care, and social security issues, to how to conduct personal relationships with friends, relatives, people at work, and lovers. The group also gets together once a month just to socialize.

In the present book, we will examine how HIV influences the HIV-seropositive person's interactions with other people, as well as the impact of HIV on the response of others to the HIV-seropositive person. Although we have introduced Ken as a person who is gay, and HIV and

AIDS have had a significant impact on the gay community in terms of how many gay males have died from AIDS, how many have been HIV-infected, and how many have known or been in a relationship with someone who was HIV-infected (see Herek & Greene, 1995; Monette, 1990; Sullivan, 1996), HIV occurs in just about any group in the population. At-risk behaviors and events that may lead to contracting the HIV infection include sexual behavior, intravenous drug use, and being the recipient of contaminated blood or blood products. In children, the transfer of the virus may occur during gestation, labor and delivery, or breast feeding. It is a fact that there are more cases of HIV/AIDS among males than females in the United States, but it is easier during penile-vaginal intercourse for HIV transmission to occur from men to women than from women to men (Kalichman, 1995). Although the greatest incidence of HIV/AIDS has been among non-Hispanic whites in the U.S. population, there is a high incidence of HIV and AIDS among persons of color (including African Americans and Hispanics). Minorities now account for more than half the new cases of AIDS reported in the United States. There has been an increase in the rate of growth of AIDS cases among minorities, but the rate of growth of AIDS cases among whites appears to be leveling off (CDC, 1996a).

The incidence of HIV and AIDS is largest in urban areas, but there are also many individuals infected with HIV in rural areas (CDC, 1996a). Although there are social, economic, ethnic, and background distinctions that affect how someone copes with HIV and AIDS, most if not all HIV-infected persons will have to confront major social issues that include who to tell about the infection, how to deal with possible disapproval or rejection, how to cope with the infection (e.g., whether to actively seek support and help from others), how to find new meaning in life under the threat of a potentially life-threatening disease, and whether to pursue life as normally as possible or withdraw from social interactions and relationships. How the HIV-infected person deals with these "social implications" of living with HIV/AIDS will depend on the personal characteristics of that person, his or her perceptions of other people, and how these others actually react.

Coping with HIV also depends inevitably on the stage of the HIV infection. Given that HIV is a progressive disease, the types of social issues HIV-infected persons may face differ if they learn about the infection: shortly after contracting the infection; during the relatively long time period when they may be symptom free; when they exhibit general and nonspecific symptoms such as persistent fatigue, rashes, night sweats, and unintentional weight loss; or when they have one or more AIDS-defining conditions (see Hoffman, 1996; Kalichman, 1995). Coping with the HIV infection will depend jointly on the personal and social resources available to the person, as well as on the stage of HIV infection and the medical and economic assets the person has to fight the disease at each stage. (It is interesting to speculate that with the availability of protease inhibitors and the trend to prescribe antiretroviral treatments shortly after HIV is contracted or with less advanced disease progression, the concept of coping with "stages" of HIV may have to be revised in the future based on medical developments; see Kahn & Hecht, 1996.)

▓ Social Aspects of Coping With HIV/AIDS

A major benefit of this book, in our view, will be to introduce concepts and original research describing how the HIV infection influences interactions and social relationships and how social behavior towards an HIV-positive person may be influenced by others' knowledge that the person is infected. The concepts and research presented in the various chapters will shed light on the everyday social concerns that someone who is HIV-seropositive (and people in their social network) may have to confront. Our approach, which focuses on the interaction and relationship aspects of living and coping with HIV, complements two other approaches that focus on (a) how to medically treat HIV/AIDS so people with HIV can live longer and with better physical quality of life and how to find a cure for the HIV infection and a vaccine to prevent it (see, e.g., Bartlett, 1996), and (b) how to devise behavioral, psychological (including clinical and counseling), and communications-based interventions aimed at reducing high-risk behaviors that might transmit HIV to others (see, e.g., Edgar, Fitzpatrick, & Freimuth, 1992; Kelly, 1995).

Although research on medical advancements in the treatment, care, and cure for HIV/AIDS, as well as on changing HIV risk behavior, will probably always predominate in the literature, the issues faced in one's social life as one copes with HIV are also important to consider.

Studying the social interaction of HIV-infected individuals is valuable per se, enabling us to understand how individuals make decisions about a number of social issues such as self-disclosure of the diagnosis to others, whether (and how) to access social support, and adjustments and/or changes in relationships with others. Focusing on social interactions in coping with HIV may also be helpful in understanding how well HIV-positive individuals are coping and in developing treatment interventions and recommendations to assist HIV-infected persons in living with the disease. Consider the following examples of the benefits of understanding the association between HIV and its social consequences:

1. Individuals who are HIV positive may become depressed as they experience physical symptoms associated with advanced stages of HIV. However, HIV-positive individuals who are relatively satisfied with informational support they have received from others are less likely to show an increase in depression over a 1-year period if they have had many HIV-related physical symptoms. The onset of physical symptoms may evoke considerable stress about what will happen next, and talking with someone who may have similar symptoms or has good knowledge about a variety of matters (such as HIV health care services, insurance personnel, or personal contacts) can be reassuring (see Hays, Turner, & Coates, 1992). If we know that satisfaction with informational social support provides a buffer against the stress associated with HIV symptoms, it would be useful, as Hays et al. (1992) recommend, to encourage HIV-infected individuals to interact with people whom they perceive as trustworthy sources of information.

2. There is research indicating that having had access to a supportive confidant (someone who can be counted on for understanding and support) and being satisfied with the quality of close relationships can decrease the likelihood of thoughts about suicide among HIV-infected individuals (Schneider, Taylor, Hammen, Kemeny, & Dudley, 1991). If HIV-positive persons are socially isolated and lonely, interventions might be aimed at overcoming their sense of social isolation to reduce the frequency of suicidal thinking.

3. There is evidence that life stressors not directly related to HIV or the progression of the disease may predict susceptibility to the development of physical symptoms associated with the progression of the HIV

infection. Evans et al. (1997) found, in a prospective study conducted up to 42 months with HIV-infected men, that for every one severe stressful event experienced per 6-month period of the research, there was a doubling of risk of early disease progression. None of the men in the study had any clinical symptoms associated with HIV disease progression at the time of their initial participation in the study. "Severe stress" as defined in the study could take nonsocial forms, such as having severe financial problems, but many of the stressful events focused on social problems that were highly threatening or unpleasant, such as the end of an intimate relationship, the death of a loved one, or being rejected by a potential relationship partner. Although there will be questions about the role of social stressors on HIV disease progression (How do these effects occur? How strong is the stress–physical symptom relationship?), the findings of Evans et al. (1997) emphasize the importance of diminishing severe stressors in the social environment of HIV-infected persons.

▓ A Social Interaction Model of Coping With HIV Infection

Figure 1.1 offers a model (building on social interaction concepts discussed in Chapter 11) that might be useful in understanding the social impact of an HIV or AIDS diagnosis. The effects of an HIV or AIDS diagnosis are associated with expectations about how long the HIV- infected person will live, availability of drugs and medications, the social status of the HIV-infected person, and his or her economic resources to deal with the infection. The impact of the diagnosis will also depend on the HIV-infected person's awareness of community attitudes and knowledge about HIV/AIDS and his or her own reactions to how the infection was contracted.

A major aspect of coping with HIV/AIDS is the possible stigma associated with being diagnosed with HIV or AIDS. HIV-infected individuals must cope with the possibility of others' disapproval, rejection, or even moral revulsion, especially if they are perceived to have contracted the disease via behaviors (e.g., male same-sex behavior, injection drug use) that are disapproved of by society at large.

The level of stigma attached to or felt by the HIV-infected person as well as that attached to HIV/AIDS as a disease will greatly influence the

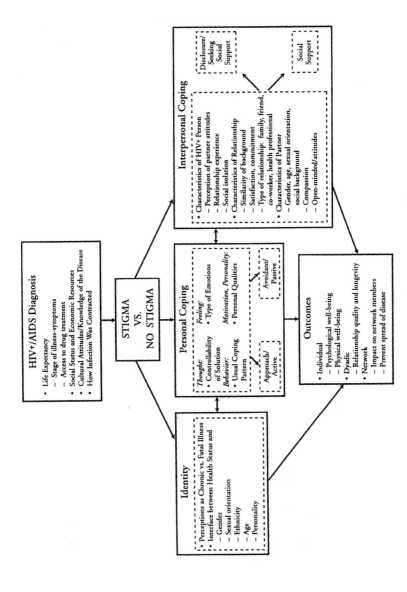

Figure 1.1 A Social Interaction Model of Coping With HIV Infection

9

infected person's identity ("Who am I?"), personal coping strategies (approach-avoidance, active-passive), and interpersonal coping strategies (e.g., disclosure of the diagnosis to others, social support seeking).

In reassessing one's identity or sense of self, perceptions of the chronicity or life expectancy associated with HIV or AIDS will influence the HIV-infected person's view of him- or herself. Furthermore, one's self-identity may be influenced by how the infection is perceived in the light of one's gender, sexual orientation, ethnicity, age, and personality characteristics.

Personal coping (how the HIV-infected person thinks, feels, and personally deals with the challenges posed by the infection) is based on perceptions of how much personal control one has in managing disease progression (e.g., via health maintenance behaviors), one's past history or usual ways of coping with stressors and threatening events in one's life, feelings evoked (e.g., sadness, optimism), and personality or motivational qualities (e.g., individual differences in desire to regain control of one's life).

Interpersonal coping concerns how the HIV-infected person copes via his or her social interactions and relationships with others, and it implies that close network members who are not infected will also need to cope with their loved one's illness. What influences the initiation of interpersonal coping (e.g., disclosure of the diagnosis and seeking social support, as well as the provision of social support by a network member) depends on the characteristics of the HIV-positive person that emerge from past experiences of and expectations about close relationships (e.g., how socially isolated and lonely do I feel, how trustworthy is a relationship partner), characteristics of the relationship between the HIV-infected person and another person(s) and/or organization(s) (e.g., perceived similarity and rapport, commitment and satisfaction with the relationship, family, friends, lover), and characteristics of the partner (e.g., gender, age, sexual orientation, compassion, open-mindedness).

The outcomes for the HIV-infected person, based on how he or she deals with social issues of stigma, self-identity, and personal and interactional coping, include effects on the individual (psychological and physical well-being), effects on his or her dyadic or personal relationships (with family, friends, intimate partners, health professionals, volunteers), and effects on the social network (which may include people at work, casual acquaintances, neighbors, and the social community).

The chapters in this book reflect, in part, the social interaction model presented here. For instance, Leary and Schreindorfer (Chapter 2) focus on the role of stigma in forming an identity based on having the HIV infection. Collins (Chapter 3) examines how the social identity of being a gay male with HIV infection affects coping and access to social support, and Rose (Chapter 4) examines similar issues of identity and psychological coping among African American gay men who are HIV seropositive. Derlega, Lovejoy, and Winstead (Chapter 8) examine the factors involved in deciding whether to disclose one's diagnosis to significant others; and Wiener and her colleagues (Chapter 10) detail the effects of disclosure (particularly in the media) on HIV-infected children. Barbee and her colleagues (Chapter 5) examine the role of social support in coping with HIV infection, including what behaviors are seen as helpful or not helpful by HIV-infected persons. Frey and his colleagues (Chapter 7) assess how organizations (based on group living in a residential facility) may provide support for people living with AIDS. Moore and her colleagues (Chapter 9) examine the effects of HIV seropositivity and the psychological functioning of partners on the quality of intimate relationships among heterosexual couples when one partner is HIV seropositive, and Omoto, Gunn, and Crain (Chapter 6) focus on how relationship experiences of volunteers working with persons with AIDS predict satisfaction and possible burnout experiences of AIDS volunteers. For a fuller description and integration of how social interaction concepts are useful in understanding how individuals cope with HIV and AIDS, see the Epilogue by Greene and Serovich (Chapter 11).

The chapters present concepts and review or summarize research that illustrates the social impact of living with the HIV infection. Implications for research, recommendations for HIV-infected persons and their significant others, and suggestions for mental and physical health professionals are also included.

We (the editors and chapter authors) hope that readers will find the book valuable as a source of information about the social aspects of being HIV infected. Our analysis and research on social interactions and relationship experiences may increase understanding of the social processes associated with coping with the disease and may promote a healthier life for HIV-infected persons and their significant others.

The Stigmatization of HIV and AIDS
Rubbing Salt in the Wound

MARK R. LEARY
LISA S. SCHREINDORFER
Wake Forest University

People who are seropositive for the human immunodeficiency virus (HIV+) report that dealing with the stigma of AIDS is one of the primary challenges and sources of stress they face (McCain & Gramling, 1992; Siegel & Krauss, 1991). Not only do they confront the trauma of learning that they have a potentially fatal disease, the prospect of a progression of painful and debilitating illnesses, and the disruption caused by recurring medical visits and hospitalizations, they also must deal with the reactions of other people to their disease and to themselves.

Recent studies of public reactions portray the extent to which AIDS is stigmatized (Kalichman, 1995). When asked how they felt about people with AIDS, 27% of the respondents in one random phone survey indicated they felt angry, 28% said they were disgusted, and 36% mentioned being afraid. Thirty-six percent of the respondents indicated that people with AIDS should be separated from the rest of society, and 21% supported the view that people with AIDS "got what they deserved." Also, the respondents clearly wanted to avoid people with AIDS: Nearly half of the respondents indicated that they would not shop in the store of someone who had AIDS, and 20% reported that they would avoid a coworker with AIDS. Perhaps most distressing, over 10% said they would even avoid a close friend who was infected. Overall, more than three-quarters of the respondents stigmatized people with AIDS (Herek & Capitanio, 1993; see also Fullilove, 1989). Such negative reactions are by no means a uniquely American phenomenon; people with AIDS evoke similar reactions in other parts of the world (Crawford, 1994; Memon, 1990). Furthermore, it is not only the general public that places a stigma on those with AIDS. Many physicians, nurses, psychologists and other health professionals also show negative attitudes toward those with the disease (Bowman, Brown, & Eason, 1994), even refusing to treat people known to be infected (Levin, Krantz, Driscoll, & Fleischman, 1995; Quam, 1990).

The focus of this chapter is on the stigmatization of HIV and AIDS. We begin with a critical examination of the *stigma* construct itself. Although it is a widely used construct in the social and behavioral sciences, stigma remains vaguely and poorly conceptualized. After offering a re-conceptualization of stigma, we examine the bases of the AIDS-related stigma and the factors that intensify and minimize the extent to which particular people with HIV/AIDS are stigmatized. The final section of the chapter deals with the psychological and interpersonal consequences of AIDS-related stigma and with the stigma management strategies of people who have HIV and AIDS.

The Concept of Stigma

In this chapter, we rely on Herek and Glunt's (1988) definition of AIDS-related stigma as "stigma directed at persons perceived to be infected with HIV, regardless of whether they are actually infected and of whether they manifest symptoms of AIDS or AIDS-related complex" (p. 886). As this definition notes, the term applies not only to the stigmatization of people with AIDS per se, but also to those with HIV. People who are not infected with HIV may also be the target of AIDS-related stigma if other people *believe* they are infected; stigmatization is based on others' assumptions about a person's HIV status, which may not jibe with reality. Also, as we will see, the AIDS-related stigma can generalize to uninfected individuals who are merely associated with someone who is known to be HIV+.

Most definitions of stigma can be traced to Goffman's (1963) semi-nal book on the topic in which he defined stigma as "an attribute that is deeply discrediting" (p. 3). According to Goffman, possessing a stigma "spoils" the bearer's social identity and disrupts social encounters be-cause both the stigmatized individual and the other participants may be distracted by the stigmatizing condition. Unfortunately, Goffman pro-vided little insight into precisely what it means for an attribute to be "discredited" or into how to distinguish "deep" discreditation from more shallow or superficial types that apparently do not involve stigma.

Jones et al. (1984) extended Goffman's definition, noting that peo-ple are stigmatized when they possess a "mark" (a deviation from a pro-totype) that has been linked to dispositions that discredit the bearer of the mark. Possessing a mark of deviance elicits an attributional process through which observers draw negative inferences about the stigmatized individual. The difficulty with this attributionally based conceptualiza-tion of stigma is that the stigmatized characteristic (that is, the mark) is not always linked to an underlying disposition that discredits the bearer. People may be stigmatized on the basis of obviously superficial charac-teristics without corresponding attributions about the stigmatized per-son's dispositions. For example, a child born with a facial deformity might be stigmatized, but not because observers make negative attribu-tions about the child; the disfigurement is inherently stigmatizing.

A third perspective on stigma was provided by Elliott, Ziegler, Alt-man, and Scott (1982). In their perspective, stigma involves a form of deviance that leads others to conclude that an individual is illegitimate for participation in an interaction. People may be judged as illegitimate interactants, for example, when they lack the ability to interact appro-priately, behave unpredictably or inconsistently, or pose a threat to other people or to the interaction itself. According to Elliott et al., once a per-son has been judged as an illegitimate social interactant, he or she is beyond the protection of social norms and may therefore be ignored or excluded altogether.

In our view, the essential feature of stigma is not discreditation, negative attribution, perceived illegitimacy, or any other type of cogni-tive response suggested by previous conceptualizations. Rather, the es-sence of stigmatization appears to be *interpersonal disassociation*. In our view, stigmatization occurs when a shared characteristic of a category of people becomes consensually regarded as a basis for disassociating from (that is, avoiding, excluding, ostracizing, or otherwise minimizing interaction with) individuals who are perceived to be members of that category.

Put simply, people are stigmatized when they are viewed as possessing characteristics that constitute a basis for avoiding or excluding them.

Consistent with previous perspectives, this conceptualization regards stigmas as originating in the shared, consensual reactions of groups of people. A personal bias against a neighbor's annoying idiosyncracies is not stigmatization. However, if a group of people share the belief that the neighbor's characteristics constitute a basis for disassociation, stigmatization is present.

▨ The Bases of AIDS-Related Stigma·

Conceptualizing stigmatization in terms of shared criteria for disassociation provides a useful, unifying framework for understanding stigma and for examining the antecedents and consequences of AIDS-related stigma in particular. If the basis of stigmatization is a propensity for social disassociation, then people are stigmatized to the extent that they possess characteristics that lead others to avoid, shun, reject, or ostracize them.

Although every society has specific criteria that determine the degree to which people are accepted and embraced versus rejected and shunned, four criteria appear to possess some degree of universality. Specifically, people are socially excluded to the extent that they

1. pose a threat to others' health or safety (by being dangerous, reckless, or contagious, for example);
2. deviate excessively from group standards (by violating morals, rules, or norms);
3. fail to contribute adequately to the welfare of other individuals or the social groups to which they belong (because they are perceived to be incompetent, irresponsible, infirm, or selfish); or
4. create negative emotional reactions in others (by being socially aversive, aesthetically displeasing, or emotionally threatening).

Presumably, people disassociate from those who meet one or more of these criteria because they perceive that such individuals pose a potential threat to the well-being of the group and its members (Baumeister & Leary, 1995).

An analysis of AIDS-related stigma in terms of this disassociation conceptualization reveals why the stigma of AIDS is so pervasive and potent: unlike nearly every other stigmatized condition, AIDS meets *all four* of the criteria for social disassociation listed above.

Threat to Health and Safety

Most obviously, people avoid those who pose a potential threat to their health and safety. To the extent that AIDS is contagious, fatal, and presently incurable, many people hesitate to interact with individuals who are known to be seropositive, despite repeated reassurances by the medical community that HIV is not transmitted by casual contact. Not surprisingly, the more contagious people believe AIDS to be, the more they desire to avoid people with AIDS (Pryor, Reeder, Vinacco, & Kott, 1989). Like leprosy in the past, HIV/AIDS possesses precisely those disease characteristics that evoke maximal fear and avoidance (Gussow & Tracy, 1968).

Given that people are stigmatized when they are perceived to pose a threat to others' well-being, people with HIV or AIDS are more likely to be stigmatized if they are known to have transmitted the virus to another person. For example, women who pass HIV to their unborn children appear to be exceptionally stigmatized, and gay men known to have infected many partners have been treated like pariahs (Dworkin & Pincu, 1993; Shilts, 1987).

Although AIDS-related stigma is no doubt partially grounded in the perceived threat of infected persons, the intensity of the stigma surrounding AIDS does not appear to be due solely to the characteristics of AIDS itself (Herek, 1990b). Thus, other factors appear to contribute to the strength of the AIDS-related stigma.

Violation of Social Standards

People are less accepting of those who deviate from their own norms, morals, and values than they are of those who conform to their social standards (Schachter, 1951). Thus, people are stigmatized when they are perceived to be members of a category that violates important social standards.

One basis of the AIDS-related stigma involves the fact that AIDS is linked in the popular mind with lifestyles that many regard as deviant, if not morally wrong. Thus, not only is the disease itself stigmatized because of its perceived threat, it is associated with groups that were already stigmatized before the outbreak of AIDS, such as gays, intravenous drug users, and, to a lesser extent, certain minority groups (Herek & Glunt, 1988). Such groups are stigmatized primarily because they are perceived as deviating excessively from prevailing standards. Because AIDS was initially identified in gay men (indeed, AIDS was originally called GRID—Gay Related Immune Deficiency Syndrome—and, more informally, the "gay plague"), HIV patients were stigmatized from the outset of the epidemic (Shilts, 1987). The finding that intravenous drug users—another group stigmatized because its behavior deviates from conventional standards—were also overrepresented among AIDS patients led to even greater stigmatization.

Presumably, deviancy serves as a basis of the AIDS-related stigma only for individuals who are, in fact, regarded as deviant, such as those who are assumed to be gay, IV drug users, or, in some cases, heterosexually promiscuous. In popular parlance, some AIDS patients, for example children and those who contracted the virus through blood transfusions, are viewed as "innocent" or "blameless" victims (Herek, 1990b). Such labels are interesting because they imply that some victims are, in contrast, to be blamed for getting the disease, presumably because they engaged in behavior that violated the standards of the perceiver's group.

Consistent with this, people view it as more stigmatizing to contract AIDS through sexual contact or drug use than through blood transfusion (Lewis & Range, 1992). In our view, this is because the person who contracted AIDS through transfusion does not meet the deviance criterion for stigmatization (although he or she may meet other criteria). This may also explain why men with AIDS are more stigmatized than are women (Lewis & Range). People are more likely to assume that a man with AIDS acquired the disease through "deviant" behavior.

The ostracism of group deviants is sometimes viewed as an unfortunate and unfair consequence of a group's enforcement of mindless conformity. When people ostracize others for characteristics, attitudes, and behavior that pose no real danger to the group, the exclusion appears to serve no function other than to avoid or punish those who are different. However, the apparent purposelessness of some instances of disassociation should not lead us to overlook the fact that those who regularly violate social standards are often a liability to the group. Violating group rules can, at best, inconvenience other individuals (as in the case of missed appointments or disruptive behavior) and, at worst, endanger their safety (as when someone falsely yells "Fire!" in a crowded theater, or when parents fail to have their children inoculated against childhood diseases). The problem, then, is not that groups disassociate from those who violate their standards but that groups sometimes disassociate from those who deviate in ways that do not, in fact, pose a threat to the group.

Contributions to the Social Good

Groups of people are also stigmatized if they are perceived as not contributing adequately to the welfare of others. Social groups place considerable emphasis on members "carrying their weight" and contributing to the well-being of the group and its individual members. Those who cannot or will not do their share are less fully accepted as full-fledged social participants than those who can and do. This criterion underlies stigmatizing reactions toward welfare recipients, homeless people, and parents who fail to pay child support. Although noncontributing members who are not able to do their share are not stigmatized as extensively as those who intentionally shirk their obligations, even those who truly cannot pull their weight are not accepted as fully as those who can. Thus, we may stigmatize physically disabled or mentally challenged people even though we know their difficulties are not their fault.

People with HIV and AIDS often cannot meet their occupational, family, and social obligations as fully as they did before they were infected. Many tire easily, must miss work for medical reasons, and, during the later stages of the disease, require assistance from other people. Even when people with HIV are, in fact, able-bodied, other people often assume that they cannot perform their normal activities. Whether their physical limitations are real or only imagined by others, people who are HIV+ may be viewed as peripheral social contributors who drain more emotional, financial, and practical resources from others than they contribute. Unfortunately, such perceptions lead to stigmatization.

Aversive Impact

People also disassociate from those who lead them to experience aversive emotions. From a simple operant perspective, we are punished for interacting with people who regularly make us feel afraid, angry, repulsed, depressed, or otherwise uncomfortable. Such a reaction is understandable, but it leads us to avoid and exclude people who cause us to feel uncomfortable through no fault of their own.

Having HIV or AIDS makes others feel uncomfortable, awkward, and anxious for many reasons (Crandall & Coleman, 1992). Aside from the fear of contagion discussed above, interacting with a person who has suffered any traumatic event can be disturbing, whether it be the death of a loved one, rape, or a paralyzing injury. Many people may be particularly uncomfortable interacting with someone known to have a terminal illness. Not only are people upset by thinking about the other person's tragedy, their uncertainty about how best to respond creates social anxiety and awkwardness (Leary & Kowalski, 1995). Some writers have also suggested that dealing with the terminally ill makes people uncomfortable because it forces them to confront their own mortality. Thus, disassociating from the AIDS patient may simply be a means of reducing one's own anxiety (Herek & Glunt, 1988). Even objects that are indirectly linked with AIDS, such as the belongings of people who are infected, may cause negative emotions and avoidance (Pryor & Reeder, 1993).

The more obvious an individual's symptoms, the more uncomfortable others are likely to feel. A person with obvious signs of AIDS such as Kaposi's sarcoma, emaciation, hair loss, or disfigurement is more likely to evoke negative reactions and is more likely to be stigmatized.

The Multiply Determined Nature of AIDS-Related Stigma

Much has been written in the popular press about the "hysteria" surrounding the AIDS epidemic, and research evidence documents the strong public reaction to people with HIV and AIDS. From the standpoint of the disassociation perspective, the extremity of this response arises from the fact that, unlike other common stigmas, the AIDS-related stigma arises from *all four* bases discussed above. For example, extremely obese people are stigmatized based on only two of the four reasons: They are perceived as violating social standards (involving both eating and weight), and they evoke negative emotional reactions in some people. They are not typically perceived as a threat to anyone else's safety, and, except in rare cases, they do contribute adequately to the social good. Likewise, unwed mothers are often stigmatized primarily on the basis of a single criterion: the violation of a social standard. Even those with leprosy, the prototypical stigmatized condition, do not meet all four criteria for stigmatization (they are usually not perceived as violating social standards). Unlike people with HIV and AIDS, few other stigmatized groups fulfill all four criteria for social disassociation.

■ Intensifiers of AIDS-Related Stigma

According to the disassociation perspective, people with HIV or AIDS are stigmatized because they are assumed to pose a threat to others, contribute inadequately to the common good, violate social standards, and/or induce aversive emotions in other people. Evidence suggests, however, that individual people with HIV/AIDS are stigmatized to varying degrees, suggesting that certain factors can intensify or minimize the degree to which the AIDS-related stigma adheres to particular cases. According to the disassociation perspective, these are factors that affect others' tendency to avoid or reject the stigmatized person.

For example, stigmatized individuals are viewed more unfavorably and treated worse if they are judged as responsible for the acquisition of their condition than if they are not perceived as responsible (DeJong, 1980; Farina, Holland, & Ring, 1966; Levine & McBurney, 1977). We see this effect operate in the instance of AIDS-related stigma: People who contracted the illness through sexual activity—particularly homosexual activity—or drug use are more stigmatized than those who contracted it congenitally or through blood transfusions (Lewis & Range, 1992). Presumably, responsibility influences the degree of stigmatization because it affects the propensity to disassociate from the infected individual.

Stigmatization is also affected by the degree to which a person's stigma increases the strain or difficulty of interpersonal interactions. Thus, people with full-blown AIDS are more likely to be stigmatized than those with latent HIV because the visibility of the disease may be more likely to disrupt social encounters and lead to avoidance (see Gussow & Tracy, 1968).

When several factors converge to increase the power of a stigma, other people's impressions of and interactions with the stigmatized person come to be dominated by the stigma, and a "master status" arises (Frable, Blackstone, & Scherbaum, 1990; Goffman, 1963; Hiller, 1982). When a person possesses a master status condition, others identify and respond to him or her as a member of the stigmatized category before other identifications are made. Being HIV+ and having AIDS are potent master status conditions. Most of us have difficulty interacting with those known to have the disease without our perceptions and behavior being affected by the fact that the person has HIV.

Consequences of Stigmatization

Learning that one has contracted a fatal illness creates immeasurable psychological distress and markedly changes how one approaches life. Relationships are explicitly and implicitly transformed, many people withdraw, and social support declines (Cherry & Smith, 1993; Collins, 1994). Along with all of the direct effects of the disease on the person's well-being, the person must deal with the stigmatization we have described. As noted, people with HIV/AIDS report that dealing with the stigmatizing consequences of the disease is one of the primary problems that they face (Siegel & Krauss, 1991).

Interpersonal Relationships

By definition, a stigma has notable implications for the degree to which others accept versus reject the individual. People often shy away from, if they do not actively shun, those who are believed to be HIV+. People often do not touch or shake hands with them, draw back from them, stare at their visible symptoms, and may even vocalize revulsion or fear (Bennett, 1990). People may be avoided by their friends, family, neighbors, and coworkers; be driven from their neighborhoods; or be fired from their jobs (Herek & Capitanio, 1993).

Because they fear these sorts of rejections, people with HIV or AIDS often conceal information about their condition from the people in their lives. As one HIV+ woman put it,

I haven't really told anyone [about being HIV+] because it's like being a leper. They really don't want to be bothered with you. It's like they totally wipe you out, and I can't afford that while I'm still healthy.[1]

Fearing rejection, people with AIDS may contribute indirectly to their social isolation. In their attempt to forestall rejection, many become guarded and preemptively pull back from their relationships. There is even evidence that the more that people feel stigmatized because of the disease, the more they miss work (Bennett, 1990).[2]

The negative reactions of family members and close friends may reflect, in part, their concerns about being stigmatized by their association with the afflicted individual (what Goffman [1963] called a "courtesy stigma"). Even if those who are close to the infected individual do not personally stigmatize HIV/AIDS, they may fear that they themselves will be stigmatized for being associated in others' minds with a stigmatized person. Such a concern is, in one sense, not unfounded. Spouses, children, family, and friends of stigmatized individuals—including mental patients, alcoholics, prisoners, homosexuals, and AIDS patients—are denigrated by association (e.g., Mehta & Farina, 1988; Powell-Cope & Brown, 1992; Sigelman, Howell, Cornell, Cutright, & Dewey, 1991). Put differently, being associated with a stigmatized person is itself often viewed as grounds for being avoided.

Unfortunately, concerns with being associatively stigmatized may lead family and friends to distance themselves from the infected person (Crawford, 1994; Lewis & Range, 1992; Stulberg & Buckingham, 1988). It may even lead family members and friends to harbor resentment toward the infected person (Stulberg & Buckingham). Because they are concerned about being stigmatized by association, the family and friends of people with HIV or AIDS, and family caregivers in particular, often go to great lengths to keep the loved one's HIV status secret (Powell-Cope & Brown, 1992).

AIDS-related stigma may linger even after the affected individual has passed away. Certain causes of death—including suicide, drug overdose, and AIDS—are stigmatized. As a result, survivors often try to conceal the true cause of a loved one's death. Because AIDS is a stigmatized death, physicians, coroners, and the news media have often been willing to oblige the families of AIDS patients, recording and reporting illnesses other than AIDS as the cause of death, thereby managing the postmortem impressions of the deceased as a favor to the family. Nardi (1990) has observed, however, that the public has gradually become aware of this practice and can now decode the euphemistic language of death certificates and obituaries. For example, many people now conclude that a young, unmarried man who is reported to have died of pneumonia, lymphoma, leukemia, or "a long illness" in fact died of AIDS (Nardi, 1990).

Not all interpersonal consequences of AIDS are negative. Some infected individuals report that their relationships with lovers, friends, and family actually deepen as other people show their explicit love and concern for the person for the first time (Bennett, 1990). In addition, some AIDS patients experience what Goffman (1963) called the "cult of the stigmatized" (p. 28) and what Herek (1990b) termed "paradoxical stigma" (p. 139). In such cases, people treat those with AIDS as if they were something special and particularly desirable. Magic Johnson and Arthur Ashe are examples of people who appear to have gained even more positive regard after it was learned that they had the disease.

Psychological Consequences

Individuals who are stigmatized for any reason experience a range of negative emotions, including depression, hostility, and anxiety (Jones et al., 1984). Being avoided or rejected by even one other person can be a painful experience; for the person with HIV, the cumulative effect of widespread social disassociation can be substantial (Baumeister & Leary, 1995; Farina, Wheeler, & Mehta, 1991). People with HIV often report feeling excluded, isolated, estranged, alienated, and lonely (Bennett, 1990; Cherry & Smith, 1993; Zich & Temoshok, 1987).

Not surprisingly, the degree to which people who are HIV+ experience a loss of social support is associated with their sense of being stigmatized. Furthermore, the degree to which people feel stigmatized correlates highly with feelings of anxiety and depression (Crandall & Coleman, 1992). Feeling stigmatized also correlates moderately with distrust of other people, although the direction of this effect is not clear. Do stigmatized people come to distrust others, or are distrustful people more likely to feel stigmatized? The greatest likelihood is that both processes occur.

People with HIV also report deep anger at others' ignorance of their condition and at others' dismissal of them (Bennett, 1990). As one person noted, "I can't put up with ignorance [about HIV]. But if someone

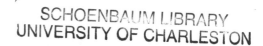

tries, and reads about it, and shows effort, then I'll talk with them about it."

Given the role that others' perceived reactions have in self-concept and self-esteem (Leary, Tambor, Terdal, & Downs, 1995; Shrauger & Schoeneman, 1979), it is not surprising that stigmatized people sometimes experience downward changes in their perceptions and feelings about themselves. People with HIV infection often assimilate society's stigmatization, perceiving themselves as contaminated and worthless (Herek, 1990b; Siegel & Krauss, 1991). At the extreme, stigmatization has been identified as one of the psychosocial stressors that may lead AIDS patients to commit suicide (Glass, 1988; Marzuk et al., 1988).

Health Sequelae

Ironically, the stigmatization associated with AIDS may actually affect the health of the infected individual in undesired ways. First, fear of being stigmatized and rejected leads some people to resist being tested for HIV (Herek & Glunt, 1988). To the extent that a delay in detection and treatment has implications for the course of the disease, such concerns can be detrimental to health.

Second, people who try to conceal their disease may experience increased stress and poor health compared to those who disclose their illness. Not only is conscious suppression of traumatic topics unhealthy (Pennebaker, 1990), failing to disclose one's illness deprives the infected person of badly needed social support. Research shows that the degree to which HIV+ people perceive social support to be available correlates negatively with symptom severity and secondary medical diagnoses (Zich & Temoshok, 1987). Additionally, to the extent that stress directly undermines the efficacy of the immune system, the distress associated with stigmatization and fear of rejection may actually encourage the progression of AIDS.

Public Policy

The stigmatization of AIDS has impeded governmental support for research and treatment (Herek & Glunt, 1988). Many public officials were initially hesitant to throw their support behind a disease that was associated with homosexuality. In one of the earliest pronouncements about the AIDS epidemic by a federal official, Secretary of the Department of Health and Human Services Margaret Heckler proclaimed, "We must conquer AIDS before it affects the heterosexual population and the general population. . . . We have a very strong public interest in stopping AIDS before it spreads outside the risk groups, before it becomes an overwhelming problem" (Shilts, 1987, p. 554). The implied messages in this early statement by a Reagan administration official are quite interesting: (a) homosexuals are not part of "the general population," (b) the government would not have a very strong interest in stopping AIDS if it were unlikely to spread outside of the risk groups, and (c) the widespread infection of certain risk groups (presumably gay men, the female partners of gay or bisexual men, and IV drug users) is not an "overwhelming problem" (Herek, 1990b; Shilts, 1987). More recently, U.S. Senator Jesse Helms argued that the federal government should not spend so much money on a disease brought on by "deliberate, disgusting, revolting conduct" ("Gingrich answers attack," 1995, p. B3). In light of such comments by public officials, it is not surprising that many AIDS patients believe that they are being purposefully stigmatized by conservative political groups (Cherry & Smith, 1993).

▦ Stigma Management

Goffman (1963) maintained that the goal of stigmatized people is to be treated as "normal." Whether or not we accept this claim as accurate, stigmatized people clearly engage in an ongoing process of stigma management to conceal, redefine, or capitalize on the fact that they possess a characteristic that other people regard as stigmatizing (Elliott et al., 1982; Jones et al., 1984; Pfuhl, 1980). As Herman (1993) observed, stigmatized people

> are not passive, powerless individuals; rather, they are strategists, expert managers, and negotiators who play active (although not always successful) roles in the shaping of deviant outcomes . . . they attempt to elicit desired reactions through their own behaviors, through the techniques of stigma management they employ, and through the expectations and images they project. (p. 324)

Passing

Many potentially stigmatizing conditions can be fully or partially concealed from other people. To the extent possible, the individual may engage in *passing:* deliberately concealing the stigmatized attribute (Goffman, 1963). Herek (1990b) suggested that most people with HIV or AIDS find it necessary to pass as healthy in certain contexts.

In the early stages of HIV infection, before symptoms of the disease become visible to other people, passing may be relatively easy. However, as symptoms develop, passing becomes increasingly difficult, and the person may devote a great deal of time and energy to concealing evidence of the disease. The infected person may try to avoid situations in which telltale symptoms would be obvious. If nausea is common after eating, the person may forego eating meals with other people who do not know he or she is HIV+. If the person has Kaposi's sarcoma under clothed areas, he or she might avoid beaches, pools, and locker rooms where the lesions will be visible. If the person tires easily, he or she must not stray too far from home or other places where it is possible to rest.

Not only does concealment necessarily restrict the person's range of activities, passing is typically stressful because the person lives in fear of detection and must provide innumerable excuses for eccentricities in his or her lifestyle (Herek, 1990b; Pfuhl, 1980). In addition, the person may be exposed to unkind jokes and negative attitudes about AIDS expressed by those who do not realize that he or she has the virus.

When evidence of illness can no longer be concealed, individuals may use remedial strategies to minimize the damage to their social identity. As their symptoms become more obvious, many people with AIDS begin to pass the disease off as other, less stigmatized illnesses—the flu, mononucleosis, or even cancer.

Disclosure and Covering

Of course, most people who learn they are HIV+ eventually disclose this fact to at least a small number of significant others, particularly after their symptoms become salient and visible (Marks, Bundek, et al., 1992). The decision to divulge that one has HIV or AIDS is often marked by extreme ambivalence and inner conflict. The person may feel a need to tell others—to obtain support, to talk through his or her feelings, or to protect the well-being of intimates and service providers—yet fear that disclosure may result in rejection. Although relatively little research exists on how people decide whom to tell, existing data show that people disclose their HIV status very selectively (see Chapter 8). People are likely to inform their partners and best friends, somewhat less likely to tell their mothers and siblings, and not likely to tell their fathers, bosses, or religious leaders (Hays et al., 1993; Marks, Bundek, et al., 1992). Presumably, such decisions are based, in part, on the degree to which others are expected to respond with acceptance or rejection to the news.

People whose HIV status is known often engage in "covering" by presenting themselves in the least offensive way (Goffman, 1963): not concealing the stigmata, but minimizing its impact on others. They may also go out of their way to convey an image of being otherwise normal despite the stigmatizing feature (what Davis, 1961, termed "deviance disavowal").

When people believe others possess negative information about them, they tend to engage in self-presentational compensation, presenting themselves very favorably in regard to other attributes (Baumeister & Jones, 1978). Thus, stigmatized individuals may try to convey highly positive impressions of themselves on dimensions unrelated to the stigma, hoping to forestall the rejection that otherwise might result.

Stigma Avowal

Finally, some people with HIV/AIDS incorporate their disease as a positive basis of their social identity. Such individuals openly avow their stigmatized condition (Rogers & Buffalo, 1974). They may even become openly and actively involved in AIDS-related causes, speaking, fundraising, volunteering, and so on. As one HIV+ individual put it,

> After I fought for 2 months to get my pride and dignity, I decided to fight for other people to prevent it from happening to someone else. It happened to me and there's nothing I can do about it, but if I can prevent it from happening to someone else, I want to do that.

Herek (1990b) suggested that people who become actively involved in AIDS groups may achieve a "level of self-esteem higher than that held by the majority of the nonstigmatized group" (p. 133). Although it may seem puzzling that a heavily stigmatized individual would not experience lowered self-esteem (Crocker & Major, 1989), people who immerse themselves in AIDS-related causes are likely to obtain a considerable amount of social acceptance by members of those groups and by other grateful people with HIV or AIDS. As a result, their self-esteem is likely to be high regardless of the reactions of the wider culture (see Leary & Downs, 1995).

▓ Conclusions

As the number of individuals infected with HIV continues to grow, more and more uninfected people will be forced to make decisions about how to deal, personally and collectively, with those who have the disease. Thus, public attitudes toward HIV and AIDS may become an even larger issue than they have been during the first decade of the epidemic.

As we have seen, the stigmatization of HIV/AIDS exacts a costly toll on the infected and uninfected alike. Real, potential, and imagined rejection create considerable distress among HIV patients and their loved ones, undermine interpersonal relationships, impede the provision of social support so badly needed by patients and their caregivers, and, all in all, make a traumatic event far worse than it would otherwise be. Stigmatization does indeed rub salt in already painful wounds.

Conceptualizing stigmatization as a process of consensual disassociation suggests that the person with HIV or AIDS suffers most not from mere denigration or prejudice, but rather from a widespread tendency for other people to avoid, exclude, ostracize, or otherwise minimize contact with them. Those who interact with people who are seropositive for HIV should be cognizant of the fact that, more than anything else, the AIDS-related stigma deprives the person who has HIV or AIDS of perhaps the fundamental psychological necessity: a sense of acceptance and belonging.

The disassociation perspective also suggests an alternative route to reducing negative reactions toward those with HIV and AIDS. In addition to simply trying to change *attitudes* toward AIDS, steps could be taken to discourage people from disassociating from those who are infected. To the extent that many people pull back from HIV+ friends and family out of uncertainty and awkwardness (rather than out of malice or prejudice), educative interventions could provide the public with guidelines that would facilitate interactions with those who are infected.

▓ Notes

1. The quotes by people with HIV are taken from interviews conducted by Val Derlega and Lisa Foster, who generously provided us with transcriptions of their interviews.

2. The stigmatization of HIV also has important implications for behavioral researchers. To the extent that people with HIV or AIDS are reluctant to disclose disease-related information about themselves, the validity of much of our data regarding the psychology of HIV infection is called into question (Brody, 1995).

Social Identity and HIV Infection
The Experiences of Gay Men Living With HIV

REBECCA L. COLLINS
RAND, Santa Monica

▓ The Implications of Gay Social Identity
for Coping With HIV Infection

AIDS is not a "gay disease." In fact, the rate of new infections in the
United States is increasing most rapidly among heterosexual women
(Haverkos & Quinn, 1995). Nonetheless, the majority of persons who
are HIV positive in North America are men who have sex with men, and
male to male sexual activity remains the primary source of new infections. The focus of this chapter is on aspects of coping with HIV that are
unique to this large segment of the infected population. Although there
are many aspects of living with HIV that are common to all persons with
the virus, the experiences of gay men depart from those of others with

AUTHOR'S NOTE: Collection of the data reported in this chapter was funded by a grant
from NHRDP Canada (#6610-1935-AIDS). I am grateful to Ruth Hahn, Lauralyn McIn-
tire, and Liann Meloff, who provided valuable assistance with coding. Special thanks are
owed to the men who shared their lives and experiences to provide the data for the study
and to their friends, partners, and family members, who also did so.

HIV in important ways. The relatively high prevalence of HIV among gays (Centers for Disease Control and Prevention [CDC], 1995b), HIV's introduction into and association with the gay male population early in the course of the epidemic (CDC, 1981), and the stigma that society imposes on homosexuality (Herek, 1990a) are factors that are specific to this population and likely to have consequences for how this group copes with the virus.

Each of these factors assumes particular importance for an individual who is HIV positive to the extent that he has developed a gay *social identity*. Social identity can be described as "those aspects of an individual's self-image that derive from the social categories to which he perceives himself as belonging" (Tajfel & Turner, 1986, p. 16). A man's sexual activity with another man does not necessarily confer a gay social identity. Rather, it is a gay man's perception that he is part of a distinct social group, and the strength of his identification with that group, that defines his social identity. A great deal of research has explored the nature and consequences of social identities. From this work, we know that group identities are largely comparative. People think in terms of the way that their group is distinct from other groups. Typically, people focus on ways in which their group is distinctly "better" than others, a process known as ingroup bias. Ingroup bias has several effects: enhancing the individual's self-esteem, enhancing his or her evaluations of fellow group members, and promoting his or her willingness to help members of the ingroup. Because ingroup bias operates among members of other groups as well, the downside is that persons outside the individual's own social category may perceive him or her relatively negatively. If, for example, I think Californians are superior to Iowans, there are likely Iowans who think the reverse. Thus, a social identity can cause one to be the object of prejudice (see Tajfel & Turner, 1986, for a review of social identity theory and research).

Because group identity is so important to self-perceptions and social relationships, it is likely to influence the manner and success with which individuals adapt to illness. This is particularly likely when the disease in question is associated with a group, as HIV infection has historically been associated with gay men in North America. Living with HIV may be especially challenging for gay-identified men, but they may also have some unique coping advantages as a result of their group membership. Both sides of the social identity coin will be explored in detail in the following pages, based on the results of an interview study of HIV-positive gay men and questionnaires sent to their friends and family members. Although the literature examining psychosocial factors in HIV is rife with studies of gay males, few investigations have looked at how their gay identity affects the ways these men live and cope with HIV infection. Thus, the interview study included some exploratory questions that allowed participants to define the issues, problems, and advantages that being gay might have conveyed in relation to their illness.

In addition to this exploratory work, a set of specific hypotheses were tested, based on social identity theory and previous studies of social responses to persons with HIV. First, I expected to find that gay men perceive their sexual identity to be an advantage in coping with HIV. As noted above, people see their groups as superior to others (Tajfel & Turner, 1986), so people probably see their group's situation or its members' ability to cope as superior to that of other people, as well.

Second, I expected gay identity and its strength to relate to the coping methods adopted by gay men. The idea that social identity facilitates active and effective coping is, in a sense, a research translation of the concept of community empowerment that has recently gained prominence. Because social identities foster self-esteem, they may help people to confront stressful situations, either by thinking about them in more positive ways ("looking on the bright side") or engaging in direct efforts to change their problems. Although there is no cure for HIV currently available, such efforts might involve activism, seeking treatment for opportunistic infections, and so on. Similarly, a positive social identity should help HIV-positive gay men to limit their use of avoidant coping strategies. Such strategies involve distracting oneself with drugs, trying not to think or talk about one's problems, or pretending a problem doesn't exist.

Third, I expected that gay identity and its strength would influence the social support that gay men receive. As I noted earlier, people are more likely to offer both emotional support and tangible assistance to members of their own group. Thus, gay men with HIV may experience more liking and acceptance, as well as more aid with everyday needs, to the extent that the gay community is part of their identities and lives.

Fourth, in examining gay identity in a broader social context and exploring the conflict between gay social identity and the social identities of those who are not gay, the prediction may be made that this conflict will influence adjustment to HIV among gay men. As noted above, social identity theory predicts that prejudice toward any given group will develop in members of other groups. Homophobia (negative perceptions of homosexuals and homosexuality) is not uncommon among heterosexuals (Herek, 1990a). Previous work indicates that homophobic individuals stigmatize gay men with HIV, viewing them as responsible for and deserving of their infection (reviewed in Crawford, 1996). Because perceptions of deservingness and blame are associated with decreased assistance to persons in need (Weiner, Perry, & Magnusson, 1988), I expected to find that gay men receive less support from those members of their social networks who are relatively homophobic.

Below, I will review and discuss the findings from this research. I will begin with an overview of the study and its design, then turn to participants' views of the issue: if and how they think living with HIV is different for gay men than it is for others infected with the virus. These subjective experiences speak to all of the study's predictions and will be discussed in this regard. They will also be used more specifically to test my first hypothesis, that participants will perceive a coping advantage in their gay identities. The remaining predictions will also be addressed with the analysis of quantitative data. I will examine the associations among items that measure gay identity strength and scales that measure participants' psychological adjustment, social support receipt, coping efforts, and their friends' and family members' attitudes toward homosexuality. In conclusion, I will discuss very briefly some ways in which the positive aspects of gay men's experiences with HIV might be enhanced and the negative aspects minimized.

A Study of Gay Social Identity and Living With HIV

The majority of the data to be reported were obtained by structured interviews of 92 symptomatic, HIV-positive gay men. Most participants resided in a large Canadian city with a visible gay community. The majority were recruited through a mailing to members and affiliates of a society run by and for people with HIV/AIDS. The organization provides AIDS-related information and services to its members and the surrounding community. Study participants ranged in age from 23 to 58; most were of European descent and without religious affiliation. Education ranged from elementary to postgraduate levels; 60% had some college training. Incomes were evenly distributed between $10,000 and $40,000 (Canadian) per year. Fourteen percent had been diagnosed HIV positive during the year previous to the interview, 50% were within 4 years of diagnosis, and the remainder had known they were seropositive for 5 to 10 years. The average participant was experiencing multiple symptoms of HIV of moderate severity and seriousness (e.g., a combination of fatigue, swollen glands, and fungal infections).

The interview was about 1½ hr in length. It covered a number of issues, including physical and psychological symptoms, coping, and social support. To assess the latter, participants identified members of their social networks and separately discussed the support received from each of them, up to a maximum of five individuals.

Additional data for tests of the homophobia hypothesis were collected directly from friends and family members. As many as three network members per participant were mailed questionnaires with the permission of the interviewee. The response rate was 76%, an average of two persons per participant. This sample was fairly similar in background to the sample with HIV. (Hereafter, the two samples will be referred to as the "significant others" and "primary participants"). Significant others had the same range of educational experiences as primary participants, although somewhat fewer had attended college (30%). Incomes ranged from less than $5,000 to more than $50,000 (Canadian) per year. Ninety-four percent were white; 52% were Christian, 10% were of other religions, 38% were not religious; 60% were male; 60% were homosexual; 13% reported that they were HIV positive. In addition to these demographics, network members provided information regarding their attitudes toward homosexuality and their tendency to stigmatize the primary participant for his infection with HIV. They also completed some other brief measures.

Respondents' Perspectives on the "Gay Experience"

Near the conclusion of the interview with primary participants, we asked them about their sexual orientation and its role in their adjustment to HIV infection:

In this study, we're looking in particular at how gay men cope with HIV infection, rather than people in general. Next, I'd like to ask you some questions about the importance of this distinction.

Respondents were asked two separate questions about their experiences:

1. In what ways, if any, do you think your experience with HIV infection has been different from that of others who have HIV and are not gay men?
2. Has being a gay man influenced the way that you coped, or how well you have coped with your illness?

To characterize responses, the author and two research assistants reviewed a set of interviews and developed a coding scheme that captured the major themes. We began with a detailed, exhaustive list of responses to the questions and then compiled related responses into larger categories and deleted from the list responses that occurred only once or twice. The final set of codes and some category exemplars are shown in Table 3.1. The author and a third assistant (who was blind to the hypotheses) applied this coding scheme to the interviews, indicating whether a respondent mentioned a particular theme or themes. Answers to the two questions were combined during coding because they tended to be quite similar. Interrater reliability, computed for a subset of 20 interviews coded by both judges, was 82%. The frequency with which each theme was mentioned is shown in the body of Table 3.1 and will be discussed further below.

In addition to applying these codes, raters made an overall judgment of each participant's response, indicating whether the respondent felt that coping was easier, harder, both easier and harder, or no different because he was gay. The majority of participants (65%) felt that living with HIV is probably easier for gay men. Not all of the men interviewed were in agreement, however. Nine percent believed that it is harder for them to deal with the illness than it is for others who are HIV positive and not gay. An equal number of respondents (9%) equally emphasized ways in which they were better off and ways in which they were worse off than others attempting to adapt to HIV diagnosis, and an additional group (12%) indicated that there were *no* differences, good or bad, be-

TABLE 3.1   Participants' Perceptions of the Impact of Gay Identity

Theme	Percent Reporting
Greater community support For example: HIV support organizations run by and for gays, gay community provides information and services, gay community is experienced with HIV, gay community accepting of HIV infection, not suspected of homosexuality like heterosexuals are, don't have to explain source of infection to others	54%
More access to others with HIV For example: have seen others cope successfully, learn about treatments from others, learn courage by seeing others die	14%
Diagnosis of HIV infection was less shocking For example: more of an expected thing, had time to think about possibility before diagnosis, don't feel like a victim like straights do, one of many instead of the "only" one	10%
Resilience to adversity developed over a lifetime For example: already know how to deal with prejudice, have developed a "survival instinct," stronger emotionally because of experience with prejudice, better at problem solving because of experience with adversity	18%
More likely to be stigmatized or blamed for own HIV infection For example: straights are seen as blameless, gays are seen to have brought HIV on themselves, AIDS is used to discriminate against gays, hemophiliacs get money from the government and gays don't	21%

tween their experiences as gay men and those of heterosexuals with HIV infection.[1] Thus, most gay men perceived their social identities as an advantage, as expected. There was some variability in response, but the disparity in the numbers reporting a clear coping advantage versus a coping disadvantage stemming from their gay identities was substantial.

Perceived Positive Consequences of Gay Identity: Being Part of a Community With High Seroprevalence Rates

Several advantages conferred by a gay social identity were noted by respondents (see Table 3.1). Of these, three were related to the high rates of seroprevalence among gays relative to heterosexuals, as was expected.

Community Support. The advantage of gay identity mentioned most often (by 54% of all respondents) was that the gay community provides a source of support for people with HIV. Participants noted that gay involvement in local HIV support organizations was very high, and that these organizations were founded by gay men and supported by funds from gay groups. Many felt that heterosexuals would feel uncomfortable using support services designed for or primarily run by gay men.

> I'm not very lucky to have this disease, but I'm very lucky in having this disease to be gay. The network of support the gay community has put together . . . if I need special tests done they'll pay for those. . . . I don't think straight people have the same access to those kinds of service and support.

> The support was greater. . . . There was a sense of coming together, you know . . . the community looked after us where the government didn't.

Another aspect of this perceived community support was respondents' perception that gays are more accepting of people who are HIV positive and that they thus received more support from their friends (who were primarily other gays) than would heterosexuals. Ironically, many suggested that heterosexuals receive less support than they do because others suspect that heterosexuals with HIV are actually closeted gays.

> I would imagine that a straight person who has HIV is just sitting there relatively alone with people close to him or her who love them, questioning things like, are they gay? Are they lesbian? And letting that factor get in the way of what they're really there for, and that's to comfort and support them.

Access to Others With HIV. Closely related to this feeling of enhanced community support was the response that being gay often means knowing a lot of other people with HIV infection. The helpfulness of contact with others who have HIV was noted by 14% of respondents. Participants felt this benefited them by providing information about treatments and legal matters, providing role models of effective coping and courage in the face of HIV/AIDS, and helping them to think about and prepare for death.

> There's more people for me to hang on to, to cope with. There's more gay men who have it so there's . . . more people for me to understand and learn from.

> I'm dealing with a larger amount of infected people who are gay . . . those who have gone through it before and those who have passed away that I've known, have given me the courage to find strength in myself, not wanting to shy away or learn to fear what I have. If anything, it just strengthens my own will—I keep going."

Thus, social support, and particularly support from similar others, may be more available to gay men than it is to others with HIV. Contact with similar others has long been thought to assist one in coping with a variety of threats (Schachter, 1959). Indeed, it has been suggested that this principle underlies the effectiveness of peer support groups (Coates & Winston, 1983). Evidence is beginning to accumulate linking participation in such groups to mental health and even physical outcomes among persons with cancer (Spiegel, Bloom, Kraemer, & Gottheil, 1989; van den Borne, Pruyn, & van den Heuvel, 1987). The present results suggest that gay men with HIV sometimes reap the benefits of affiliating with similar others without having to attend support groups. As a result of HIV's high prevalence among gay men, many gay men have access to people with HIV through their preexisting social networks. This may provide a strong advantage in coping.

It should be kept in mind, however, that if being gay means having a network of sick friends, it also means that many people close to the participant will be or have been lost to AIDS. The pervasive bereavement experienced by many gay men in the era of HIV/AIDS can, obviously, be a stressful experience (Folkman, 1993; Levine, 1992; Martin, 1988). This stress may outweigh any benefits conveyed by having coping models. Nonetheless, bereavement was not the focus of present participants' thoughts: Those who mentioned that their friends were ill or had died referred to what they had learned from these others, not to their own distress. It is significant that participants found this positive meaning in their experiences of loss. Perceptions that stressful life experiences contribute to one's "life-education" are an important part of coping with trauma (Taylor, 1983). Whether the derivation of meaning from loss allows people with HIV to come through their bereavement experiences better adjusted than they would be if they faced their illness alone is an important question that future research should address.

Expecting the Diagnosis. Participants' perceptions that they have greater community support and greater access to similar others than do heterosexuals are likely to be a result of HIV's relatively high prevalence among gays. A third category of response also stemmed from the unequal distribution of HIV prevalence across heterosexual and gay populations: A small subset of participants (10%) felt that it is easier for gay men to cope with HIV because gays feel less singled out by fate.

> Because I was homosexual, I was prepared to have the disease. I had given it 6-8 years of thought since it had come out and been pounded into our systems.

> Oh to them [heterosexuals], it would be a shock . . . It would be like having a rare form of something, you know, like "Why me?"

One of the more devastating aspects of illness can be the knowledge that one is vulnerable to major negative events. According to theory, people rely on a set of assumptions about themselves and the world that allows them to function and feel secure (Janoff-Bulman & Frieze, 1983). These assumptions consist of the beliefs that the world is just and that bad things do not happen to good people. Disruption of this set of beliefs, one's "assumptive world," is thought to be a common consequence of major illness. When something bad (e.g., a diagnosis of illness) does occur, the individual is forced to conclude either that he or she is a bad person or that negative events are random and uncontrollable.

Evidence partially supports this hypothesis. In one study (Janoff-Bulman, 1989), undergraduates were asked about the major stressful events that had occurred in their pasts; they then completed a scale measuring assumptions concerning justice and beliefs about one's own self-worth. Those students who had had a victimizing experience saw the world as more threatening and themselves more negatively than did the typical student, consistent with the predictions of just world theory. However, a subsequent study of cancer patients indicated most of them held more *positive* views of themselves and the world than they had held prior to their illness. Ancillary analyses indicated that, to the extent they engaged in active coping, participants were able to prevent their world assumptions from shattering and actually enhance their positive belief systems (Collins, Taylor, & Skokan, 1990). Their efforts to change or rethink their situations and to seek social support led them to the conclusion that they had come relatively intact through something they would have thought psychologically devastating. Thus, they felt more invulnerable than ever.

In the present study, some participants thought that they had adapted to HIV better than heterosexuals had because they had expected to be infected by the virus. This suggests that assumptions about the world are also preserved by having advance warning of a threat. Perhaps knowing that one is at risk for an illness allows one to cognitively prepare for its diagnosis, putting coping mechanisms into play before it actually occurs. If so, this has implications for the (psychological) advisability of newly available technologies like genetic testing for cancer risk.

Perceived Positive Consequences of Gay Identity: The Effect of Lifelong Prejudice

In addition to the advantages conferred by being part of a larger community affected by HIV, many participants (18%) felt that they had benefited from their sexual identities more directly. Over the course of their lives, participants argued, they had developed personal strength and coping ability as a result of being gay, and this had helped them to confront HIV and AIDS better than others might.

> Because as a gay man, through life, we've always had to work and struggle much harder than anybody else who has not had to deal with discrimination from fellow students, family. . . . And so these things, all these things build a strength that a lot of other people don't have.

> Well, life has always been a fight . . . so this is just another fight.

This fascinating finding, that coping with prejudice prepares one to deal effectively with other forms of adversity, was not expected. However, such a response to lifelong stigma and prejudice has been discussed in the research literature before. In his pioneering book *The Nature of Prejudice*, Gordon Allport (1954) conjectured that individuals and groups who experience prejudice develop certain personality characteristics as a consequence. These traits begin as coping mechanisms,

Allport argued, but eventually become stable aspects of personality. This is exactly the sort of effect that gay men in the present study reported experiencing. However, Allport contended that insecurity, self-hate, and denial of group membership were the likely result of prejudice. The present participants indicated that prejudice had had positive effects on their personalities, that they developed resilience and strength as a consequence of their persecution. Their perceptions certainly make sense. Strategies developed to deal with one stressor, prejudice, may help one cope with negative events of all kinds. Future work should attempt to determine when, why, and in what ways people derive benefit from prejudice, rather than being damaged by it.

Perceived Negative Consequences of Gay Social Identity: Homophobia and Blame

Not all of the men interviewed felt that they were better off because they were gay. Nine percent believed that living with HIV is harder for them than it is for those with the virus who are not gay. Ironically, given the resilience result just noted, all of these men felt that coping with HIV was more difficult because they were doubly stigmatized, first by having HIV and second by being gay. In addition, many of those who felt they were, in balance, better off than heterosexuals with HIV still reported problems with being stigmatized. In total, 21% of participants suggested that they were the objects of a double stigma. Some described specific instances of rejection. One respondent who left his job after his diagnosis described the lengths to which his supervisor went to avoid shaking his hand on the day of his departure. He felt the man's fear of contagion would not have been there, or at least would not have been as strong, if the respondent had been a woman with HIV or a hemophiliac. More typically, references to stigma were made in general terms.

> Because I'm gay . . . it's harder. If I was straight I could be the poor innocent victim of a blood transfusion or the poor mixed-up junkie. . . . I got what I deserved as far as the straight community is concerned.

> [People say AIDS is] the gay plague and, you know, God damnation type thing . . . instead of saying it's just a disease doing what diseases do—affecting everybody.

These claims are supported by what is now a wealth of studies addressing the correlates and causes of HIV-related stigma. According to a recent review (Crawford, 1996), 17 studies have documented a correlation between negative attitudes toward homosexuality and negative reactions to persons with HIV/AIDS. Although somewhat indirect, this suggests that gays may be especially stigmatized by HIV. Better evidence is provided by studies that have tested whether a gay man with HIV/AIDS is responded to more negatively than others with HIV infection. These studies have found that gay men are more likely to be blamed or stigmatized than persons described as hemophiliac or heterosexual. Gays were more likely to be held responsible for their infection and people were more likely to limit their social contact with gay men than others with HIV (Fish & Rye, 1991; St. Lawrence, Husfeldt, Kelly, Hood, & Smith, 1990; Weiner, Perry, & Magnusson, 1988). Thus, respondents' perceptions of stigma are almost certainly veridical.

Other Perceptions of Gay Identity and Its Consequences

A few respondents (9%) were uncertain where the balance between good and bad fell in their experience as gay men and emphasized equally ways in which they might be both better and worse off than others with HIV infection. An additional group (12%) felt there was no difference between their experiences as gay men and what others faced in coping with HIV infection. The latter group said things like

> You got HIV, you got HIV. It doesn't make any difference whether you're gay or straight, male or female . . . I mean, we all came from straight families. We all have to tell straight families.

> There's no stereotypes. In each person it's radically different. There are very few similarities except for the fact that we tend to get the same diseases and ailments.

This group was typically unable to expand upon this perspective, viewing it as self-evident that gay men are no different from anyone else (hence, there are no codes associated with this response in Table 3.1). Some participants noted that who they have sex with has nothing to do with coping with illness. The social identity aspects of life as a gay male, such as the stigma and the community support noted by others, were clearly either not a part of these men's experience or were viewed as irrelevant to the task of coping with HIV. This finding underscores the importance of distinguishing among different subgroups in studies of gay-identified men. Some gay men consider their sexual orientation a central part of their self-definitions and their lives; others see it as unnoteworthy or even feel negatively about being gay. "Internalized homophobia," negative perceptions of homosexuality in a gay man, may predict difficulty adjusting to HIV infection, because it may lead to self-blame (Herek & Glunt, 1995). A lack of strong self-definition as gay may also hinder coping in that it may limit use of the community support noted by participants. Exploring the impact of differences in the strength of gay identity was one goal of the next set of results I will present.

Relationships Between Gay Identity Strength and Adaptation to HIV: Adjustment, Coping, and Social Support Advantages

The following results also serve to verify and expand upon participants' perspectives regarding the relationship between being gay and coping with HIV. Studies of the introspection process indicate that people's inferences regarding the causes of their thoughts and feelings are often erroneous (Nisbett & Wilson, 1977). Thus, respondents' reports about the adaptational impact of gay identity may not be entirely veridical. Instead of reflecting actual experience, respondents' reports may be a part of the coping process in themselves. Research regarding the phenomenon of "downward social comparison" indicates that people often say or think they are advantaged, even if it is not true, to feel better about their illnesses. Perceptions that others are worse off may make people feel less victimized by their own situations (Wood, Taylor, & Lichtman, 1985). Thus, it might be true in the present study that, for example, gay men with HIV get more support from AIDS service organizations than do heterosexuals, or it might be that this perception is an illusory one, used by gay men with HIV/AIDS to reassure themselves that their situation is not the worst one possible.

If the reports of respondents are not veridical, they are still important in providing insight to the subjective experience of gay men with HIV. They would also remain relevant, under such circumstances, to the question of how gay identity influences adaptation to HIV. Gay identity may serve as a convenient hook on which to hang one's hat of relative advantage, facilitating the downward comparison process. Nonetheless, to fully understand the process by which social identity contributes to coping (i.e., whether the benefit it provides is relatively objective or subjective), it would be desirable to test the impact of gay identity in a way that does not require respondents to infer cause and effect, as do the introspections reviewed above. Separately measuring identity and its hypothesized impact and then examining their correlation constitutes such a method, and I used this approach in the next set of findings I will present. This tactic will also allow us to explore differences between gay men in the ways that they view their social identities and in the strength of their gay identities. Both the content and strength of gay identity may have a critical impact on how it affects coping with HIV.

To permit examination of these issues, participants were asked to rate, along a continuous scale, the strength of four different aspects of their gay identities. The four items used reflect the central components of social identity as outlined at this chapter's outset (Tajfel & Turner, 1986). Following an introductory statement that conveyed the concept of a social identity, respondents reported the extent to which (a) being a gay male was central to their self-image, (b) the gay community was a part of their lives, (c) gay males, as a group, are different from other people, and (d) they were proud or happy to be a gay man. Responses were made on a four-point scale ranging from one (*not at all*) to four (*very*). Mean item ratings were 3.00, 3.03, 3.15, and 3.49, respectively, indicating that the average participant had a moderately strong gay social identity.

One way in which social identity was expected to be of assistance is by influencing the coping strategies chosen by seropositive gay men. A revised version of the Ways of Coping Inventory (Folkman, Lazarus, Dunkel-Schetter, DeLongis, & Gruen, 1986) was used to assess respondents' coping behavior, so that its correlation with identity could be tested. The coping inventory employed contained six subscales (complete information concerning subscale development and reliability is included in Collins & Di Paula, 1997). *Cognitive avoidance* included items like "I wished the situation would go away" and "I had fantasies about how things might turn out." *Behavioral avoidance* was measured with items like "I tried to make myself feel better by eating drinking, smoking, or using drugs" and "I avoided being with people in general." *Distancing* is a method of coping similar to cognitive avoidance but suggests a refusal to react to the illness rather than an avoidance of it. It was measured with items including "I didn't let it get to me" and "I made light of the situation; refused to get too serious about it." *Self-presentational coping,* a subscale new to this study (see Collins & Di Paula, 1997, for details), involves efforts to hide distress from others and might be considered the social equivalent of distancing. It included the items "I tried to appear in control of the situation" and "I put up a happy front when around others." Each of these subscales was considered an avoidant or negative method of coping, and scores on them were expected to be inversely related to gay identity.

Two active forms of coping were also measured: seeking social support and focusing on the positive. The seeking support scale included the items "Talked to someone who could do something about the problem" and "Talked to someone about how I was feeling." Focusing on the positive was measured with items like "I rediscovered what was important in life" and "I was inspired to do something creative." These active coping scales were expected to relate positively to gay identity.

Gay identity was also expected to relate positively to social support receipt. Several measures of support were collected. Emotional support from friends, that is, the extent to which friends showed the participant he was loved or cared for, was measured by averaging scores on the Social Support Questionnaire—Short Form (Sarason, Sarason, Shearin, & Pierce, 1987) across all friends described in the interview. Instrumental support from friends (the extent to which friends helped with meals, shopping, and other chores) was measured with a modified Activities of Daily Living Scale (Schulz, Tompkins, Wood, & Deekers, 1987).[2] Network size and the number of new friendships respondents directly attributed to their HIV diagnosis (e.g., people met through HIV support organizations) were also assessed.

Coping Results. The associations between the measures of gay identity and those of coping were examined first, by computing correlations between each identity item and each coping subscale. It was expected that participants with a strong gay identity would cope more effectively, and results were supportive of this idea. Participants reporting higher levels of gay pride less often used cognitive ($r = -.31$) and behavioral ($r = -.24$) avoidance to cope with HIV. They also hid their distress from others less often ($r = -.19$) and were somewhat less likely to use distancing ($r = -.17$). Gay pride was unrelated to the two measures of active coping: seeking social support and focusing on the positive. Correlations and significance tests for all the identity and coping variables are shown in Table 3.2.

As this table indicates, associations between the other three identity items and coping were largely nonsignificant. Greater participation in the gay community ($r = .25$) and seeing gay men as different from other people ($r = .20$) were both associated with focusing on the positive aspects of one's illness. Seeing gay men as different from others was also related to distancing ($r = .20$). Because 24 correlations between identity and coping were examined, these scattered associations should be interpreted with caution. However, the findings concerning pride and coping were consistent. Gay pride, but not other aspects of a gay social identity, appears to be an important resource for adapting to HIV infection. Although pride was not strongly related to active coping, it was related to less use of passive or avoidant coping methods. Avoidant coping is typically inversely related to adjustment, so this negative relationship suggests that gay pride is adaptive.

Social Support Results. The importance of gay pride to coping with HIV infection was also demonstrated in the correlations computed between the gay identity items and the measures of social support. Participants who were more proud or happy to be gay reported significantly more emotional ($r = .21$) and instrumental ($r = .19$) support from friends. They also had somewhat larger networks of close friends and family ($r = .17$) and had formed more new relationships that they attributed to their HIV diagnosis ($r = .20$). Those who felt that the gay community was an important part of their lives had also formed a greater number of new relationships as a result of their diagnosis ($r = .25$). None of the other social identity items were significantly associated with any form of social support.

Thus one specific aspect of social identity, a feeling of pride in being gay, played a role in the social support experiences of gay men with HIV infection. This sense of pride is arguably the core of the social identity concept, which emphasizes the bolstering of self-esteem through group membership, as I have noted. Participation in the gay community may also play a part in social support, apparently by maintaining or improving the size of social networks following HIV diagnosis. It has been ar-

TABLE 3.2 Correlations Among Gay Identity Items, Coping Behaviors, and Social Support

	1	2	3	4	5	6	7	8	9	10	11	12	13	14
Gay Identity														
1. Central to self-image	**91**													
2. Community involvement	.33*	**92**												
3. Distinct group	-.04	-.04	**92**											
4. Gay pride	.38*	.20*	-.02	**90**										
Coping														
5. Cognitive avoidance	-.07.	.07	-.04	-.31*	**75**									
6. Distancing	.05	-.01	.20*	-.17#	.37*	**75**								
7. Behavioral avoidance	-.08	.10	.06	-.24*	.61*	.29*	**75**							
8. Self-presentation	-.13	.02	.14	-.19*	.44*	.57*	.21*	**77**						
9. Positive focus	.09	.25*	.20*	-.09	.03	.20*	.20*	.02	**75**					
10. Support seeking	-.01	-.02	-.01	-.06	.05	-.11	.24*	-.05	.53*	**75**				
Social Support														
11. Emotional support	.10	.09	.11	.21*	-.11	-.06	.04	-.21*	-.01	.13	**89**			
12. Instrumental support	.05	-.03	.06	.19*	-.04	.00	.11	.03	.14	.10	.37*	**89**		
13. New relationships	-.16#	.25*	-.15#	.20*	.05	-.10	-.03	.00	.24*	.17#	-.03	-.08	**91**	
14. Network size	.14	.14#	.08	.17#	.00	.20*	-.09	.10	.11	-.04	.04	-.10	.08	**92**

NOTE: Numbers in bold print (along the diagonal) indicate the number of participants with data for each item or scale.
#p < .10; *p < .05.

gued by some that disclosure of HIV infection often results in the disintegration of relationships. Involvement in the gay community may help compensate for such losses, if they occur, by facilitating the acquisition of new social ties to replace those that are broken following HIV diagnosis. However, the lack of strong associations between community involvement and other aspects of social support suggest that the relationships formed in this way do not provide emotional or tangible assistance to gay men with HIV.

The other two aspects of identity that were measured, feeling that gay men are different from other people and feeling that being gay is central to one's identity, were unrelated to any aspect of social support. It may be that feeling one's group (gay men) is different from others facilitates relationship formation with other gay men but isolates one from the larger social world, resulting in no overall benefit in terms of social support. It is less clear why the centrality of sexual orientation to identity was unimportant. Perhaps some participants who viewed being gay as self-defining saw this identity negatively (the correlation between pride and centrality was .38; see Table 3.2). Presumably, defining oneself negatively would have a negative impact, and this might wash out any effects of having a positive self-definition in the aggregate analyses conducted.

Adjustment Results. The relationships between gay pride and two important psychosocial resources, coping behavior and social support, suggest that gay identity strength may also be associated with psychological adjustment, as was predicted. The Symptom Checklist–90 (Derogatis, 1977), which measures states of anxiety, hostility, and depression, was administered verbally at the outset of the interview. When correlations between scores on each of these subscales and the four gay identity items were computed, their pattern was much like that obtained for coping and social support. That is, gay pride was significantly associated with less anxiety, $r(90) = -.18$, $p < .05$, and less depression, $r(88) = -.20$, $p < .05$, and the other identity items were uncorrelated with either measure. None of the items, including gay pride, was related to hostility scores.

Further analysis indicated that the relationship between gay pride and adjustment may be mediated by (i.e., operates through) gay pride effects on coping behavior and social support receipt. Statistically controlling for the coping and support variables virtually eliminated the inverse associations between gay pride and negative emotion. This suggests that pride in one's gay identity facilitates adjustment to HIV infection by influencing these other variables. Gay pride improves the social resources available to gay men and reduces their reliance on negative coping strategies, which in turn fosters well-being. Of course, the collection of data at a single point in time makes it impossible to confirm that these relationships are causal, but results are consistent with this hypothetical chain of events.

Summary of Identity Strength Findings. The present findings are consistent with those of the few studies of coping with HIV that have included gay-related factors among their predictor variables: Community involvement has a tenuous relationship to adaptation to HIV infection, and gay pride has a relatively strong relationship to adaptation. In one study, Lackner and colleagues (1993) found that a variable tapping participation in the gay community predicted less depression at a later time point. However, community participation was among the weaker predictors of depression, and several measures closely related to the concept of community involvement were unassociated with adjustment. Lackner's results suggest, as the present study does, that the adaptational advantages of community involvement may be weak or inconsistent.

In contrast, the few studies that have looked at gay pride in relation to coping with HIV have consistently found positive associations between pride and effective adaptation to illness. Nicholson and Long (1990) found that negative attitudes toward homosexuality among HIV-positive gay men were related to avoidant coping, and negatively related to adjustment. They also found that homophobic attitudes were inversely related to active coping. Wolcott, Namir, Fawzy, Gottlieb, and Mitsuyasu (1986) found that positive attitudes toward homosexuality were correlated with both social support satisfaction and psychological adjustment among gay men with HIV. Finally, the importance of gay pride was demonstrated in a study by Herek and Glunt (1995). They found that gay men coping with the threat of HIV and AIDS were better adjusted when they had a positive gay or bisexual identity and fewer negative attitudes toward their own homosexuality. Each of these studies used a somewhat different sample and a different operationalization of gay pride, yet all reached a similar conclusion: Gay pride helps gay men to cope with adversity.

These findings complement the present participants' reports of their subjective experiences as gay men, adding to these reports some specificity regarding the aspects of gay identity that influence adaptation to HIV and the processes through which gay identity influences adjustment. However, we have so far considered only the up side, the ways in which being gay can be helpful in living with HIV infection. Previous studies of homophobia and stigma, as well as the perceptions of participants in the present study, suggest that gay men's experiences with HIV are also worse in some ways than those of heterosexuals with the virus. This is considered next.

Homophobia, Blame, and Adjustment to HIV

In their responses to the open-ended questions, participants indicated that the stigma attached to HIV infection is enhanced when one is gay. Even many of the participants who felt they were, on the whole, better off than heterosexuals reported that stigmatization was a problem for gay men with HIV. This is the negative side of social identity: It often results in derogation of one's group by people who are part of another social category (Tajfel & Turner, 1986).

As noted earlier, a number of studies have demonstrated a relationship between prejudice against gays and HIV stigma. However, virtually all of these studies have relied on similar methods. Typically, college students or health care providers are given a written description of a person with AIDS. After reading the vignette, participants are asked to make a judgment regarding the likability or the culpability of the person described. This vignette method is a useful tool for studying the factors that influence people's perceptions of others. However, vignette studies can be limited in their generalizability. The participants in such studies are asked to judge people about whom they have little information and with whom they share no relationship. It is questionable whether the same factors that evoke stigma in this situation would influence someone asked to judge a longtime friend or family member who has been diagnosed with HIV infection. In the context of a wealth of information regarding the character and the previous health behavior of someone with HIV—someone whom you care about—homosexuality may be of no importance, even to persons who are homophobic. If so, the added stigma confronted by seropositive gay men may be specific to their interactions with strangers, casual acquaintances, and policymakers.

The roles of homophobia and stigma within close relationships were tested as part of the interview study. Because the results have been reported in detail elsewhere (Collins, 1994), I will review them only briefly here. As noted early in this chapter, participants' friends and families participated in the study by filling out a mailed questionnaire. This questionnaire included measures of homophobia (Bouton et al., 1987) and of HIV-related stigma (Kelly, St. Lawrence, Smith, Hood, & Cook, 1987b). The homophobia scale assessed extent of agreement with items like "homosexuality is immoral." The stigma measure was a scale commonly employed in the HIV literature and taps the perception that a person with HIV is deserving of and responsible for his or her illness. The correlation between network members' homophobic attitudes and their stigmatizing perceptions of participants was examined as part of a larger test. In the model examined, stigma was treated as an outcome variable, and the contributions of HIV status, homophobia, sexual orientation, and the interaction between the latter two variables were simultaneously explored. Such a test reveals the impact of each of the predictive factors while statistically controlling for the others.

The result revealed a positive association between homophobia and stigma. That is, a negative attitude toward homosexuality among loved ones was associated with a tendency to blame their gay friend or family member for becoming infected with HIV, just as such attitudes have related to blaming strangers in other studies. However, there was an important qualification to this effect. The interaction between homophobia and sexual orientation was also statistically significant, indicating that the relationship between phobia and stigma depends on one's sexual orientation. Follow-up tests showed the pattern of this effect, revealing that homophobia and stigma were associated only among heterosexual members of gay men's social networks. The homophobic attitudes of other gays were unrelated to blame.

Thus, it seems that gay men with HIV face stigma on several fronts. They may be blamed for their illness not only by society, but by some of the persons with whom they share close relationships. This stigma clearly adds to the burden of coping with HIV. It is interesting that in participants' narratives concerning the impact of being gay, reports of stigmatization seldom included friends or family as the source. Such experiences were occasionally noted at other points in the interview, particularly when respondents were asked to describe unhelpful things that their friends or family had done since their diagnosis (see Chapter 5 for similar data), but not during the gay identity questions. It may be that, when thinking about experiences with stigma, the reactions of society are more salient or more important than those of one's intimates. Alternatively, having lived with someone's homophobia for some time prior to HIV diagnosis (as would likely be true of a friend or relative), an unsupportive reaction by this individual may seem part of one's general life experience rather than one's specific experience with HIV. It was only HIV that participants were asked to discuss in relation to their gay identities.

An unexpected result also turned up in the analyses of stigma. There was a significant effect of sexual orientation, indicating that gay network members tended to stigmatize men with HIV more than their heterosexual friends and family did (Collins, 1994). Although no prediction had been made regarding this issue, a finding of *less* blame among other gays might have been expected, if anything. Indeed, the simple correlation between sexual orientation and stigma was nonsignificant, indicating that gays are not typically more blaming of persons with HIV. However, given the statistical approach used, which controlled differences in gay and heterosexual network members' levels of homophobia, gays held more stigmatizing attitudes toward their friends or relatives with HIV. Thus, a gay man with HIV will find that, between a gay friend and a heterosexual friend, his gay friend will be more blaming of him for his illness *only* if the two friends hold equivalent attitudes toward homosexuality. Even with this qualification, the finding that gays can be more blaming of persons with HIV than are heterosexuals is surprising. Two related theories concerning the manner in which people attribute the cause of negative events may explain it: defensive attribution (Shaver, 1970; Walster, 1966) and just world theory (Lerner, 1970).

Both theories argue that people reduce their fear of negative events by attributing responsibility for negative outcomes to the events' victims. As noted earlier in this chapter, people maintain a sense of personal safety by believing that bad things don't happen at random. By blaming victims' behavior for their problems, or seeing victims as deserving, people can conclude that, as long as they don't make the same mistakes themselves, they will not have similar experiences. Because this attributional pattern is self-protective in nature, any factor that promotes feelings of personal threat should enhance the motivation to blame victims.

Consistent with this, a review of 22 studies of defensive attribution (Burger, 1981) found that victims who were more similar to the person making an attribution were more likely to be blamed by him or her. Tests of just world theory have produced similar results (Lerner & Miller, 1978). Such an effect may be responsible for the elevated levels of HIV-related stigma observed among gay men whose levels of homophobia approximate those of heterosexuals. These men may be inclined to attribute blame for HIV infection to other gays out of a desire to see infection as avoidable for themselves.

Another possibility should also be considered. It may be that gay men see HIV infection as blameworthy not because of a self-protection motive but because sexual risk reduction has been strongly promoted in the gay community. A cornerstone of health behavior interventions is response efficacy—convincing people that if they take the recommended health precaution, they will be safe from risk (Rosenstock & Kirscht, 1979). People who are successfully convinced that they can avoid HIV themselves may believe that anyone who contracts the virus could and should have avoided infection. In short, risk reduction campaigns may inadvertently increase the stigma associated with HIV infection. Because gay men have been the target of most of these interventions, they may tend to be more blaming than heterosexuals.

The relationship between sexual orientation and blame that was obtained in this study had not been anticipated, and no data were collected to test either of these interpretations, so they remain speculative. It is also important to keep in mind that, at the bivariate level (i.e., when homophobia was not controlled for statistically), there *was* no relationship between the two variables. Heterosexuals were just as blaming as gay social support providers. Only after homophobia was statistically controlled for did an association between sexual orientation and stigma emerge.

The final question to be considered in this chapter is the impact of stigma on gay men's adjustment to HIV infection. Are those who are stigmatized by loved ones worse off psychologically? I examined this question in further analyses of the stigma data (Collins, 1994). The results revealed that persons whose support networks stigmatized them were, indeed, more poorly adjusted than others. This relationship between stigma and well-being was partly a function of stigma's inverse relationship to the emotional support provided by heterosexuals. To the extent that heterosexual friends and family members felt that a study participant was to blame for his HIV infection, they provided less support, and this reduction in aid partially accounted for the association between stigma and poor adjustment.

▓ Conclusions

The data presented in this chapter suggest a number of ways in which gay men with HIV both benefit from and are hindered by the social identity that their sexual orientation potentially conveys. Some of the results merely substantiate what has long been argued, that gay men are more stigmatized than others with HIV. However, the present findings take this idea somewhat farther. Gays with HIV are blamed for their illness not just by the general public, but by their heterosexual friends and family members who hold negative attitudes toward homosexuality. Even more disturbing is the unexpected finding that other gays may sometimes also blame them for their illness. The basis for this finding could not be determined, but two explanations were offered: that culpability for the illness was attributed defensively, out of fear of HIV, and that risk reduction campaigns may inadvertently promote stigma. Both possibilities clearly warrant further examination, should this finding prove replicable.

Given the toll that HIV/AIDS has taken on gay men as a community and as individuals, it would be inappropriate to uncover such effects without offering some ideas about how to rectify the situation. The reduction of stigma is a daunting challenge: Many years of psychological research and intervention and decades of public policy have failed to eliminate other forms of prejudice from American society. However, some approaches have shown promise and might be considered in future research. For example, Monteith (1993) gave college students feedback regarding their scores on a measure of homophobia. By making participants aware that they are more prejudiced than they had thought, she was able to reduce their prejudiced responses to gays on another laboratory task. The effectiveness of this strategy may be limited to reducing stigma among persons who are already relatively low in prejudice. However, Monteith has also identified a strategy that is effective with persons high in prejudice: making them believe their prejudiced opinions are not normative (Monteith, Deneen, & Tooman, 1996). Monteith's strategies need to be tested in the field, using a broader population and methods amenable to influencing large audiences, but they show promise. If they can be successfully applied to the reduction of HIV stigma, the present study suggests, gay men with HIV will be better able to adjust to their illness and more likely to obtain the social support they need.

In the meantime, many men are benefiting from their gay social identities. Indeed, the findings presented in this chapter indicate that gay identity does HIV-positive men more good than harm. Living with prejudice all their lives has made these men resilient, able to deal with new challenges in effective ways. It has also resulted in a strong, supportive community that mobilized quickly in response to HIV/AIDS and continues to provide assistance. Finally, those who take pride in their sexual orientation are able to marshal vital coping and support resources to assist them in living with HIV. For some participants in the present study, this pride was externalized through the symbols and events of the gay community—the Gay Pride parade was mentioned often. For others, gay pride was something internal, a satisfaction with themselves. One participant put this particularly well: "I don't go waving a flag or anything but . . . proud? Very."

Nurturing this pride and fostering it in other gay men, through community programs, public policy, and a reduction of gay prejudice in the general population, may be one of the more important ways that gay men can be aided in their efforts to not just live with HIV, but live well.

▨ Notes

1. Positive, negative, and neutral responses sum to only 95% because four of the interview tapes were inaudible. The more specific aspects of participants' experiences (e.g., feeling resilient, feeling stigmatized) sum to more than 95% because many gave responses that fit more than one category.

2. Family support was also measured but was not examined in these analyses. The association between family support and gay social identity is likely to be complicated, involving issues of homophobia addressed later in this chapter. Because family members are less freely chosen than friends, it is more likely that family members disapprove of the participants' sexual orientation (i.e., are homophobic). Friends may evidence some small level of homophobia, but it is likely that persons who feel very negatively toward homosexuality would not have gay friends.

Searching for the Meaning of AIDS
Issues Affecting Seropositive Black Gay Men

SUZANNA ROSE
University of Missouri–St. Louis

I'm waitin' on time; time ain't waitin' on me.
—Michael Anthony Caboose Hayes, Jr.

Black gay men who are seropositive, like others facing life-threatening illness, must learn to cope with the initial knowledge they are infected, as well as continue to adjust over the course of the disease. Coping is difficult physically, emotionally, and spiritually, as indicated by Michael, the 30-year-old seropositive Black gay man quoted above.

AUTHOR'S NOTE: The author would like to express her deep appreciation to Ron McLean, Erise Williams, and Blacks Assisting Blacks Against AIDS, St. Louis, for helping to make this study possible. Many thanks are also extended to the participants who generously shared their stories, including Sebastian, Cedric, Mr. N, Michael Anthony Caboose Hayes, Jr., Desiree DeMornay, Betty Boo, Curt Tarkington, Tony Thomas, Marcus Williams, and four anonymous participants.

I found out I was HIV positive about 5 years ago. I was really devastated . . . shocked. [It] has really changed my whole, entire life. I mean, it's nothin' you can get rid of. It's something you think about each and every day. . . . It is a bitch. You never forget it for a minute. It is with you 24 hours a day. It's with you in your sleep. It never goes away. It changes your life in ways you don't even know, ways you didn't even know you could. . . .

And it's nothin' to play with. It's *nothin'* to play with! Goin' to the doctor is nothin' to play with. Takin' medication is not nothin' to play with. You just deal with it the best way that *you* know how. . . . Life is meant to be a joy. I didn't know in my life how *bad* I took advantage of life doin' everything I wanted to do. With it [HIV] creepin' up on you— it's not nothin' to play with *at all*! Because you never know when you're gonna get sick. You never know when you might die. . . . It's not a joke. It's a bitch. It is *not* a joke. I've been livin' with that for almost 6 years.

People who experience life-threatening or traumatic events theoretically undergo a cognitive readjustment process that has been proposed by Taylor (1983) as focusing on three themes: a search for meaning in the experience, an effort to regain mastery over the event and one's life, and a desire to enhance one's self-esteem despite the personal setback. Specifically, the search for meaning involves an effort to understand the significance of the event, including what caused it and what meaning life has now. Mastery is reflected in concerns the individual has about how to keep another or similar event from happening and how to manage the current event. The self-enhancement theme represents efforts to find ways to feel good about oneself again, often by comparing oneself with others who have worse problems.

The cognitive adaptation process of interest in the present chapter is the search for meaning. The search for meaning is regarded as a primary human motivation within humanist-existential perspectives (Frankl, 1984; Lerner, 1980). This view implies that sense *can* be made of the negative outcome. Traumatic events are believed to initiate a search for meaning among survivors because they often shatter people's views that the world is understandable and orderly (Janoff-Bulman, 1992). Finding meaning in life's misfortunes represents an adaptive coping strategy that has been shown to restore or maintain psychological and physical health among many types of trauma survivors, including cancer patients (Taylor, Lichtman, & Wood, 1984) and incest victims (Silver, Boon, & Stones, 1983).

One critically important source of the meaning attributed to any traumatic event derives from its sociocultural context, including widely held beliefs about the particular traumatic event (Lebowitz & Roth, 1990). Also relevant is the extent to which stigmatization of the person affects coping (see Chapter 2). In addition, whether an individual is able to derive meaning from the trauma is believed to be determined by the interaction of multiple forces, including the person's life history, his or her personal resources, the specific characteristics of the traumatic event, and social discrimination and poverty (e.g., Horowitz, 1979; Kalichman, 1995; McCann & Pearlman, 1990).

The first goal in the present chapter is to explore how the sociocultural context inhabited by seropositive Black gay men potentially affects their search for meaning. Second, quotes from in-depth interviews with a small group of seropositive Black gay men will be used to illustrate themes related to the search for meaning; these quotes will be compared to those found in previous research on seropositive White gay men (Schaefer & Coleman, 1992; Schwartzberg, 1993).

▨ Sociocultural Context of AIDS for Black Gay Men

Understanding the sociocultural context of AIDS is important for both the prevention and treatment of HIV infection among Black gay men, who are in a relatively high-risk group for contracting HIV. Estimates indicate that one of every 33 Black men between the ages of 27 and 39 in the United States may be infected (Rosenberg, 1995). Among Blacks, male same-sex activity is the most common form of transmission of AIDS/HIV cases, including 39% of actual AIDS cases and 32% of cases of HIV infection (Centers for Disease Control and Prevention [CDC], 1996a). Male-male sexual contact combined with injection drug use is the source of exposure for another 8% of AIDS cases and 5% of HIV infections. In contrast, about 36% of AIDS cases and 22% of HIV infections among Black men were reported to be due solely to injection drug use, and only 6% of AIDS cases and 9% of HIV infections were attributed to heterosexual contact (CDC, 1996a).

Although male-male sexual contact clearly represents a significant risk factor for HIV among Blacks, public awareness and prevention campaigns virtually have ignored Black gay men. Homophobic attitudes have been linked to the perception originally held by ethnic minority groups that AIDS was a White man's disease (Peterson, 1995; Peterson & Marin, 1988). Denial of the existence of homosexuality within ethnic minorities has been noted for Black, Asian, and Hispanic American communities. Homosexuality tends to be equated with a rejection of fundamental cultural values within these groups and may be stigmatized as "immoral," "disgusting," or "sick" among ethnic minorities even more so than in mainstream White culture (Chan, 1995; Icard, 1986; Mays, Cochran, & Rhue, 1993; Savin-Williams, 1996; Tremble, Schneider, & Appathurai, 1989). For Black Americans specifically, social norms have required that homosexuality not be explicitly acknowledged (Peterson, 1992, 1995). Consequently, HIV transmission in Black communities has been primarily regarded as a problem among injection drug users and their heterosexual partners, which was also identified as the transmission route to infants and children (Peterson, 1995). HIV-related programs in the White community neglected Black gay men as well. White gay men have organized very strong community responses to HIV in urban areas; however, little attention has been placed on Black gay men by most of these efforts (Peterson, 1995).

The stigmatization of homosexuality by ethnic minority cultures contributes to the development of a dual identity for gay men and lesbians of color (e.g., Chan, 1993; Espin, 1993; Loiacano, 1993; Marin, 1989) and is likely to have important consequences for how Black gay men cope with AIDS. To be gay is to reject traditional family roles and cultural values and, subsequently, to be perceived within the ethnic minority community as having assimilated oneself into White culture (Loiacano, 1993). Thus, ethnic minority individuals who openly identify themselves as gay or lesbian may risk losing the support of their community. On the other hand, to identify oneself as Asian, Hispanic, or Black may require negating one's gay identity within the family and community. A dual identity is also reinforced within White gay communities, where Black gay men and lesbians may obtain support for their sexual orientation but may be stigmatized due to their race (Icard, 1986; Savin-Williams, 1996).

The stigma associated with homosexuality among Blacks has one other significant consequence. Black men who have engaged in male-male sexual contact have been found less likely than other groups to classify themselves as homosexual (e.g., Stokes, McKirnan, & Burzette, 1993). Some of these men prefer to classify themselves as bisexual; others may label themselves as heterosexual, particularly if they assume the traditional masculine role in their same-sex contacts such as being the inserter during oral or anal sex. Discomfort with one's homosexual or bisexual behavior has been found to be associated with high-risk sexual behavior among Black men (Mays, Cochran, & Bellinger, 1992; Peterson et al., 1992). Thus, the stigma of homosexuality may influence Black gay men to take fewer precautions than others to protect themselves or others from HIV infection. In addition, Black men who label themselves as gay may represent only a subset of the population of Black men who have sex with men.

A seropositive HIV status adds an additional stigma with which Black gay men must contend. People with HIV/AIDS report that one of the primary problems they face is dealing with the stigmatizing consequences of the disease (Siegel & Krauss, 1991). Because a stigma is "an attribute that is deeply discrediting" (Goffman, 1963, p. 3), stigmatized individuals are viewed as possessing characteristics that others use to devalue them and that are used as a basis for avoiding or excluding them (see Chapter 2). The consequences of AIDS-related stigma include social isolation from friends and family, negative emotions such as depression, hostility, and anxiety, and symptom severity (Chapter 2). Thus, seropositive Black gay men must cope with the trauma of having a potentially fatal disease as well as occupying three stigmatized identities—being seropositive, Black, and gay.

An important issue to explore for understanding the experience of seropositive Black gay men is how occupying multiple stigmatized identities affects coping with HIV. Research has not yet focused specifically on this topic. Instead, the available research on stigma documents prejudice based on the assumed singleness of identity. Race, gender, sexual orientation, and disability have all been studied separately, but seldom has there been a study dealing with a cross-section of these. Each stigma has been associated individually with negative interpersonal and economic outcomes (Crocker & Major, 1989), so a possible consequence of multiple stigmas may be to intensify stress and impair functioning. However, the effect of bearing several stigmas may not necessarily be additive. Some research indicates that members of stigmatized groups may develop ways of reacting to prejudice that are self-protective and that continue to maintain high self-esteem (Crocker & Major). Consequently, in at least some cases, it may be that prior experience with one stigma would make it easier to cope with additional stigmas. For example, in Chapter 3, Collins reports that gay pride and involvement with the gay community provided White gay men with a unique resource that positively affected adjustment and coping with HIV.

One factor that may affect coping with multiple stigmas is whether they are visible or, if not, whether they have been disclosed. Because race is a visible stigma, stereotyping, prejudice, and discrimination against Blacks is likely to cause many Black gay men to identify more strongly with the Black community than the White gay community (Icard, 1986; Johnson, 1987). In contrast, being gay or having HIV (unless one is in the later stages of AIDS) are concealable stigmas. Subsequently, many Black gay men may choose to conceal their gay identity within the Black community. Concealment of homosexuality has been found to increase the likelihood that Black gay men will engage in high-risk sexual behavior (Peterson et al., 1992). Concealment of a seropositive status may also be chosen as a way of avoiding rejection by prospective sexual partners, as well as family (Hoff, McKusick, Hilliard, & Coates, 1992). Those who conceal both identities may eventually be forced to disclose both simultaneously, increasing the stressfulness of the disclosure. As with other gay men and seropositive individuals, disclosure may lead to loss of support from family and friends. However, Black gay men with HIV risk losing community support that provides a buffer or refuge from racism, as well.

Other sources of stress that have been identified as having an impact on coping with HIV include economic hardship due to racism, a history of sexual abuse, and trauma due to bereavement. Economic hardship such as lack of employment opportunities due to racism or sexual abuse history has been associated with high-risk sexual behaviors. Individuals who have been prevented from obtaining a sense of belonging or achievement through economic means might realize these motives through increased or indiscriminate sexual activity (Fullilove, Fullilove, Haynes, & Gross, 1990). Gay men who were sexually abused as children or adolescents have been found to more frequently use psychoactive and injection drugs, attempt suicide, engage in unprotected anal sex, and receive mental health counseling and hospitalization than nonabused men (Bartholow et al., 1994). Bereavement due to HIV has been shown to increase the number of mental health problems among gay men, including sleep problems, recreational drug use, depression, and demoralization (Martin, 1988). The number of losses and distress resulting from loss may have adverse effects on the immune system, as well (Kemeny et al., 1994). Additional stressors that have not been studied but that reasonably might affect coping include child abuse, domestic violence, or other victimization.

The church is one institution within the Black community that has the potential for helping seropostive Black gay men deal with multiple stigmas and the trauma of HIV. Evidence indicates that Blacks tend to use religion more often than Whites to cope with a variety of problems, including HIV (e.g., Jackson, Neighbors, & Gurin, 1986; Jenkins, 1995). Research also shows that religious coping potentially contributes to a sense of well-being, ameliorates distress, and helps people to reinterpret the meaning of stressful life events in a positive way (e.g., Pargament et al., 1990; Reed, 1987). However, religious teaching has also been identified as a source of intolerance toward people with HIV and homosexuals (Bell, 1991; Worth, 1990). To the extent that intolerance is a part of church teaching within the Black community, Black gay men with HIV will be deprived of an important source of support. Given the high rates of HIV among Blacks, it may be especially crucial for Black religious organizations to lead the way in developing grassroots advocacy and support programs for people with HIV. In some communities, Black churches have been slow to respond to this need (Shelp, DuBose, & Sunderland, 1990).

The White gay community is a second potential source of support for seropositive Black gay men, one that has been limited in the past by social prejudice and institutional discrimination against Blacks. Discrimination by White gay and lesbian communities has been ranked as one of the most persistent problems ethnic gays and lesbians experience (DeMarco, 1983; Mays et al., 1993; Morales, 1983). If ethnic gays and lesbians are accepted by the White community, they may be expected to place their sexual identity foremost in their lives and to minimize their racial concerns (Savin-Williams, 1996). In regard to AIDS outreach, some urban White gay communities have only recently begun to target Black gay men and other ethnic groups specifically (Peterson, 1995). As a result, the resources of the White gay community may not be readily available to seropositive Black gay men.

In sum, seropositive Black gay men inhabit a unique sociocultural context that could reasonably be expected to affect the cognitive readjustment process believed to occur when individuals experience a traumatic event. Aspects of the sociocultural context that were introduced as potentially playing a role in Black gay men's search to understand the meaning of an HIV positive diagnosis included how the stigma associated with homosexuality and HIV within the Black community affects Black gay men's identity, the effect of multiple stigmatizations on coping, the impact of other sources of stress such as racism, and the response of Black churches and the White gay community to the problem of HIV among Black gay men. The preceding discussion suggests that, due to sociocultural influences, the search for meaning among seropositive Black gay men may not be directly parallel to that of White gay men, who more often have been the target of empirical research.

▓ The Search for Meaning

In this section, we will describe themes present in the search for meaning among a small group of seropositive Black gay men. Two studies have focused specifically on how HIV affects beliefs about the meaning and value of life; both used in-depth interviews with mostly White gay men (Schaefer & Coleman, 1992; Schwartzberg, 1993). The intent here is to compare the sample characteristics and responses of Black gay men participants with those of White gay men studied previously to provide greater understanding of how seropositive Black gay men cope with HIV.

Schwartzberg (1993) focused on the effect of HIV on gay men's beliefs about the world and themselves, using qualitative analyses of interviews with 19 participants who were recruited by word of mouth, by flyers, and by the researcher personally. Sixteen of the participants were White, 2 were Black, and 1 was Hispanic. Ages ranged from 27 to 50 years (median age was 40 years old). Almost all were economically stable and well educated. Fourteen had a college or graduate degree and 4 of the remaining 5 had some college education.

Schaefer and Coleman (1992) examined the specific meanings associated with HIV among 20 seropositive White gay men who were recruited from an HIV clinic at a midwestern university medical center. All were White, between the ages of 20 and 55 years (median age was 36 years old), and well educated. Sixteen had some technical or college education and 5 had a bachelor's or master's degree. The sample was economically stable and employed in middle-class occupations such as service, technical, management, and professional jobs; some owned small businesses.

In contrast, the 13 seropositive gay men interviewed by the author in the present study were Black, younger, less affluent, and less educated, reflecting a different sociocultural context. All participants identified themselves as gay and had sought treatment or services at one time from Blacks Assisting Blacks Against AIDS (BABAA) in St. Louis, Missouri. Individuals were invited to participate in the research through BABAA directly, were referred by a private therapist who was connected with the organization, or learned about the research through word of mouth. The participants ranged in age from 20 to 40 years (median age was 28 years old), and all identified themselves as gay. The group was predominantly working class or lower middle class as reflected by their education and occupation. Three had completed some high school, 2 were high school graduates, and 7 had completed some college. Only 1 was a college graduate. Participants' occupations included clerk (fast food, store, or government), waiter/food service, janitor, truck driver, electrician, machine operator, graphic artist, floral designer, and female impersonator.

It is reasonable to speculate that the material and psychological circumstances for the Black gay men prior to HIV diagnosis were significantly more limited than those of the White gay men sampled by Schwartzberg (1993) and Schaefer and Coleman (1992), given their current socioeconomic differences. If so, Black gay men's ability to find meaning in the experience of being seropositive may be expected to have been adversely affected by those limitations. Repeated traumatization has been shown to result in emotional reactions such as fear, anxiety, depression, self-esteem disturbances, anger, guilt, and shame, as well as behavioral problems like aggressive and suicidal behavior, substance abuse and impaired social functioning, and interpersonal problems (McCann, Sakheim, & Abrahamson, 1988). Most of the Black gay men who were interviewed described numerous experiences with economic hardship, psychological trauma, or drug use that may have been less common among White middle-class gay men. For example, parental child abuse led to two of the Black gay men being placed in foster homes as children; two others were raised by relatives. Four men reported having been sexually abused as children. Two repeatedly had attempted suicide before testing HIV positive. Five participants indicated that they had been addicted to drugs (alcohol, cocaine, crack, and marijuana) before learning of their HIV status. Seven men described having been in at least one physically abusive relationship in the past. Two had been the targets of serious gay bashings involving sexual assault and multiple injuries requiring hospitalization. Thus, it is possible that these events would have inhibited or forestalled the search for meaning among the seropositive Black gay men interviewed here.

The current study was exploratory in nature, similar to the research by Schaefer and Coleman (1992) and Schwartzberg (1993). The basic question guiding it was, "How does HIV affect the meaning of life?" Views of the self, others, and race were explored in this context. The goals of the research were to identify (a) the global meaning of HIV for participants, comparable to Schwartzberg (1993); and (b) specific meanings of HIV for Black gay men, similar to Schaefer and Coleman (1992). The semistructured interviews with seropositive Black gay men focused on the following areas: the sociocultural context surrounding diagnosis, including family and community support and relations with the White gay community; impact on relationships; openness about sexual orientation; current adjustment and self-image; benefits and costs of HIV; and views of the future. Questions were also asked about other psychosocial stressors that might affect coping (e.g., poverty, drug use, sexual abuse, AIDS-related bereavement). Interviews were conducted at the participant's home or a venue of his choosing and generally lasted from 1 to 2 hours. Interviews were tape-recorded and transcribed. The methods and results are described and compared to Schwartzberg (1993) and Schaefer and Coleman (1992) below.

▓ Global Meaning of HIV

The method used by Schwartzberg (1993) to investigate the global meaning of HIV was similar to that employed in the present research. Schwartzberg asked open-ended questions focusing on the participant's gay identity; relationships; HIV-related changes in sexual behaviors and attitudes; psychosocial adaptation to HIV; issues of mortality, death, and illness; medical concerns; experiences with grief and bereavement; AIDS in the gay community; spirituality; and substance use. The interviews in Schwartzberg's study (as well as in the present study) were then examined to see what general trends were revealed in participants' ability to find meaning in HIV. Participants' affective presentation, consistency of the material reported, and recurrent themes over the course of the interview were also used to assess general patterns.

Four global patterns of meaning were identified by Schwartzberg (1993) and used to classify the mostly White participants, including high meaning, defensive meaning, shattered meaning, and irrelevant meaning. Those who ascribed high meaning to HIV were individuals able to transform the despair of a potential "death sentence" into an opportunity for personal growth. These men felt that HIV was, paradoxically, a thing of value, a chance to discover an inner potential or strength of which they had not been aware. White gay men in the defensive meaning group spoke positively of HIV as a catalyst for personal growth, but the growth seemed superficial. Often, they viewed HIV as a punishment, a representation of HIV that was at odds with their boasts of great personal change. They gave the impression that their belief in their transformed self would not sustain them in a crisis. Participants in the shattered meaning group did not have a meaningful framework for their HIV infection. They had asked "Why me?" but no satisfying answer was found. They were embittered and depressed and also suffered from unresolved grief due to bereavement from AIDS losses. Those in the irrelevant meaning group perceived HIV as not having had much impact on how they understood their world. They insisted AIDS had not changed them in any way. They compartmentalized their infection so that it was not a dominant aspect of their identity.

In the present study, following Schwartzberg (1993), interviews were examined to answer the question, "What overall patterns were there in participants' ability to find meaning in HIV and AIDS?" Global trends in participants' responses to AIDS were examined, including the consistency of statements, themes recurring over the course of the interview, and the participant's emotional state. The four categories of meaning derived by Schwartzberg were used by the author to group participants' responses: high, defensive, shattered, and irrelevant.

The Black gay men were distributed about evenly across the four categories, similar to Schwartzberg (1993). A profile from one participant per category s given below to illustrate each category.

Group 1: High Meaning (4 of 13). Similar to 7 of Schwartzberg's (1993) 19 participants, 4 of the seropositive Black gay men were able to transform the enormous upheaval of learning of their HIV infection into an opportunity to shape their life in a more meaningful direction. The ability to find high meaning appeared to transcend the participants' actual health status. One of the 4 was asymptomatic, 1 had had several medical indicators of HIV (e.g., thrush, bronchitis) but was stable, and 2 had more serious medical conditions. Each of the 4 believed that HIV was something that tapped a deeper or more spiritual part of themselves, providing them with a calling that required them to help or love others.

Marcus (31 years old) explained, "I am a strong believer in fate," as he recalled having his fortune told in 1984 by a woman who said, "You're gonna get a disease from loving a man." In 1988, another omen occurred when a stranger remarked to him, "I see you in the ministry in a grey suit. An AIDS ministry." Marcus responded to these and other similar incidents by asking God "not to use me in AIDS," but went on to state,

> God often uses you in the way you fear most . . . [but] it seemed it was inevitable. I would have to accept the call. If I didn't tell others about my situation [after learning about his HIV status], I would truly die. At that moment I understood what healing truly is. I had to let go of any animosity I had toward people. I felt like, "This is my time. This is my chosen path."

Being able to give to others granted the men a sense of worth that compensated for any real or imagined failure, hardships endured, self-blame, or dependency on others due to HIV. For 2 of the men, supportive relationships were present before HIV diagnosis; in fact, 1 (Mr. N) had cofounded BABAA before he was infected. For the other 2, the experience of giving and receiving love did not occur until after HIV. A profile from this group is presented in Table 4.1A.

Group 2: Defensive Meaning (4 of 13). Four Black gay men who were grouped in the defensive meaning category appeared to be struggling with strongly contradictory or ambivalent feelings about HIV, comparable to 3 of the men interviewed by Schwartzberg (1993). These men indicated that being HIV positive had resulted in significant personal growth; at the same time, their responses conveyed considerable anger, regret, and fear. They wanted to believe good would ultimately outweigh the negative aspects of HIV, but simultaneously expressed serious doubts

TABLE 4.1   Illustrations of Four Categories of Meaning for Coping
With HIV/AIDS Among Black Gay Males

A. High meaning group profile

"As I grew up, I never got love," recalled Maurice Anthony, age 20, as he described a family history of severe physical and sexual abuse that left him a ward of the state at a young age. "I looked for love in places that got me to where I am now—that led me [before age 13] to an older man, a 42-year-old schoolteacher who sang in the choir. . . . I did all kinds of things with him unprotected—anal sex, hard, painfully. He would put a gun to me. He physically and sexually abused me. . . . He told me he loved me. No one had ever told me that, even my mother. . . . [I believe] this man gave me AIDS. . . .

"I learned [I was HIV positive] at the age of 15, the same time Magic Johnson was on TV. . . . I was wonderin', 'Could this be me?' I got tested that day. [After being diagnosed] I thought my life was over. This is *it*. This is my life sentence. I thought I had one day [left]. I was afraid to go to sleep. . . . I went through a lot of denial. I've tried suicide on several occasions. A cord around my neck. Pills. I thought, 'I've been raped and abused, how much worse can life be?' But it *was* worse! I had to be constantly educated on this [HIV]. I would look in the mirror and think, 'Filthy. Dirty.' I'd call myself names. 'How can anybody love me? You're so ugly and with this disease, how can anybody love you?' It's the support that BABAA, my two best friends, and my gay family have given me that's changed my life. My mother is even part of my support now. . . .

"[Due to HIV] I've gotten a chance to see life for what it really is. I've helped a lot of people. I was on TV recently for a program on teens and AIDS. Will I go to heaven, or go to hell because I'm gay? My life has flashed before me on several occasions. I was just in a car accident. . . . I realized I could die of anything, not just AIDS. I used to be as weak as a tree limb, but now I'm strong as steel. . . . I want to be like Will, my mentor [at BABAA]. I'm a support for a lot of people. Look at how I've come from point A to point F. You *can* do it!"

B. Defensive meaning group profile

"Let me tell you up front and be as honest with you as I can," remarked Michael Anthony Caboose Hayes, Jr. (30 years old). "I'm not scared of dyin'. I'm not. I have *lived* my life. I may not turn 31. I've lived my life and had myself to back me up and I've *loved* it. All the people I've been involved with, I love them. I never realized life was so fuckin' wonderful. That you can be anything that you want. . . . I mean, I can't believe my whole fuckin' life has changed just that fuckin' quick. . . . Life before, it was very active. Very active. Sexually active, too. I did some things I regret. Had sex, you know, stuff like that. Then on top of that, usin' drugs—cocaine—doesn't really help. I was strung out for a while and brought myself back together. . . .

"I have put myself together. I really have done a great job fixin' myself. I'm a witness. I go to a lot of seminars, do a lot of work for the community. I love it. This is my life now. This is the way I have to live my life. Because I have HIV—that don't mean I'm *dead*! I'm not dead! I'm still out here doin' great things, tryin' to educate young people. . . . I may not live to see 40, 45, 50. But that's not my business. I live each and every day as if it's the last day!

"The only thing positive about HIV is that you know what you have. You see stuff more now than other times in life. You focus on your whole ability to be a person. As a Black gay man, you look at people differently—you see what's inside of them. Your emotion changes. You get real in depth with somebody—the inner self of somebody. . . . It's so damn sickening that it had to take a motherfuckin' disease for somebody to bring out their inner self to you!

"Some change is for the worse, but I don't consider it to be a problem. I've had a very good life. I don't have remorse or hate anyone. . . . [but] it *is* a bitch. It's really hard. You might be doin' something else, then suddenly there it [HIV] is in your head. My friends will ask me, 'What's wrong?' But it won't go away. It never goes away."

C. Shattered meaning group profile

"I'll never forget getting tested [for HIV]," said the 23-year-old Black gay man who asked that his stage name as a female impersonator, Desiree DeMornay, be used. "It was November 17, 5 years ago. . . . It's been an uphill battle asking, 'Why did God do this to me? What did I do that was so wrong?' . . . I was in a daze. I thought I must be asleep. . . . I'm gonna wake up. . . . [but] I'm not dead or sick. It doesn't inhibit me from doing what I want to do. It's been hard because things about my body has changed— discolored skin, swollen glands, rashes. . . . The mental is worst. I really want to die, [but] if I kill myself, I'm afraid of that will happen to me [in the afterlife]. Are there things in my life I would do differently? [pause] But I've enjoyed everything I've done. . . . All through grade school and high school I was a straight A student. I received numerous awards and certificates of merit. I was listed in the newspaper for being in the honor society. I always loved the stage. . . . I went to NYU [New York University for a while. . . . There have been a lot of men in my life. I was very popular.

"I can't imagine life without HIV. To me, HIV is a lesson from God. It's not because he wants to kill everybody off. He wants to teach us the meaning of life. It would be a boring life if nothin' was ever wrong—no colds or cancer. . . .

"I'll probably live to be 28, hopefully, if I keep takin' care of myself. . . . It's the deterioration of the body that scares me. My T-cell this week is under 200. I'm really scared. This is the point at which I could catch pneumonia and I could be gone. I'm afraid of germs, fungi. I'm constantly cleaning—door knobs, the phone. I haven't worked for about a year except as a female impersonator three or four times a week. It's tiring me, but I get enjoyment from it. I enjoy people saying, 'You look wonderful.' I've been pretty depressed lately. When I'm sad, I'll put on my makeup and clothes at home and escape. . . . Desiree is a different person—she's sultry, sexy, and glamorous. Desiree is my best friend. . . ."

D. Irrelevant meaning profile

"I've known for three years that I was HIV positive," explained Melvin (age 40). "The doctor who told me said that 85% of the people who get tested didn't want to know [their results]. That was me. I didn't want to know. . . . My doctor said, 'Melvin, if your T-cell is less than 500, you must take AZT. If it's under 200, it's AIDS.' When she said, 'It's 76,' I almost fell off the chair! She said, 'If you need 1000 and you have 76, you won't be here long.' [pause] I dropped a few tears. But I thought, 'If you live this rambunctious a life, what do you expect? . . .

(continued)

TABLE 4.1   (continued)

"I didn't go into hiding or act ashamed. I've always lived to be a blessed person. I wasn't promised any years to live when I came out of my mother's womb. It could be 40 years. It could be 80 years. I never knew. I've been in the military. I've gone to college. I've been blessed. . . . It [HIV] didn't change anything. . . . I didn't feel sorry for myself. I won't have a problem mentally dealin' with the symptoms. . . . I didn't blame anyone. I'm a level-minded person. It's done. I can't blame anyone for my own sexual activities. I wouldn't have gone to bed with someone who was [HIV] positive, but of course, I didn't know.

"I go through loneliness. That's all that bothers me. Nobody wants to be alone. Loneliness takes its toll on me, but it doesn't bow me down. . . . I don't go through any emotional stress about the virus. I don't even think about it. Why should I think about it? . . . I don't think AIDS is a terrible illness. If you're a diabetic, you're on dialysis two, three times a week. If you have cancer, you've got to take chemotherapy. I have a different illness.

"Until God decides to call my name and it's time to go, I'll be ready. I believe in my spirituality. I don't care how sick you may get, you're not goin' nowhere until the Lord says, 'Time to go.' He doesn't seem to be ready for me. He wakes me up every morning to get ready for work."

that HIV was anything more than a tragedy. They were also uncertain of their ability to meet the challenge of future health-related crises. Johnny Jones, with a low T-cell count of 5 at 28 years of age, indicated that he would not allow anyone to put a time limit on his life, which he viewed as "a celebration." However, his assertions of "feeling good" and "I don't worry about things" were interspersed with anxiety about medical symptoms such as numb feet and lightheadedness that threatened his sense of stability. See Table 4.1B for a profile from this group.

Group 3: Shattered Meaning (3 of 13). Three of the Black gay men could not derive any significance from HIV; they viewed it as leading to loneliness and loss, as was the case for 3 of Schwartzberg's (1993) participants. They also tended to blame themselves for getting HIV either through an active sex life or because their desire for love and attention was so great they did not act to protect themselves. All indicated they were quite depressed and presented as such. The men in this group, more so than the other 3, had difficulty confiding their HIV status to family and friends. Two were not explicitly out to their family as gay men, but both claimed their families "knew." The social isolation of this group was related to feelings of loss. One 22-year-old man who requested the pseudonym Tony Thomas said,

> I tested positive when I was twenty. . . . I didn't tell my family. I didn't want to put any of my burdens on them. . . . I can't imagine telling my mother at all. My main wish is to outlive her. I know how her [blood] pressure is under stress.

A profile from a participant classified with the shattered meaning group is presented in Table 4.1C.

Group 4: Irrelevant Meaning (2 of 13). Two of the Black gay men indicated that HIV had little impact on their self-concepts, relationships, or worldview. Four of Schwartzberg's (1993) 19 participants were placed in this category. These men asserted that HIV was just something that had happened to them, but they felt it could easily have been something else instead. They compartmentalized HIV in their life and did not see it as an identity; it was an illness like any other. Both men were functioning well emotionally, even though one was disabled to the point of needing a wheelchair to get around. This man, Dwight (age 35), said,

> At first I was a little shocked [to learn of his HIV status]. After that, I said to myself, "Life goes on." . . . I look on the bright side. I look to the man upstairs. No use cryin' 'bout it 'cause you already got it. Eat healthy.

The men in the irrelevant meaning group did not appear to be defeated. Their approach was quite practical. Both took responsibility for the sexual practices that led to infection and felt the important issue was to go on from there. Dwight explained, "I don't blame myself—but I do fault myself. I didn't really know to be safe." The other man, Melvin (age 40), had a philosophical approach, "You live this lifestyle for so many years, what do you expect?" Table 4.1D shows a more in-depth profile of a participant from this group.

In sum, the four categories proposed by Schwartzberg (1993) proved to be a useful system for describing how seropositive Black gay men responded to HIV. It is important to note that although the four categories are presented as distinct, participants' responses tended to overlap categories to some degree, similar to Schwartzberg's findings. Thus, the actual complexity of response is diminished. Furthermore, the ability to find meaning was an ongoing process for each individual as he confronted new aspects of the disease. However, the categories served as a useful template for understanding the ways people struggle to make sense of AIDS.

Several other similarities between Black gay men and White gay men studied by Schwartzberg (1993) are also significant. First, most of the Black gay men had also been able to find some good in their HIV diagnosis, most often with regard to the personal growth or connections with others it had enabled them to achieve. Second, as for White gay men, no consistent characteristic could be discerned that governed an individual's placement in a certain category. For example, there was no relationship between health status and the ability to find meaning. Those whose infection had progressed to AIDS were represented in all four categories. AIDS-related bereavements also did not affect categorization, because all of the men had suffered bereavement due to AIDS. All had lost a friend, 3 a partner, 2 a sibling or close relative, 1 a partner due to an AIDS-related suicide, and another 3 were currently involved with partners who were in the later stages of AIDS. Third, Black gay men spoke with animation and at length about their attempt to find meaning in their situation, as did the White men, suggesting that the search was relevant to coping with trauma. Most importantly, the quest did not appear to be circumscribed for Black gay men by numerous previous economic and psychological adversities. If anything, their response to the challenge of HIV appeared to be met with a quiet dignity that belied their pre-HIV behavior and hardships. In fact, several of the seropositive Black gay men asserted that they valued very little about themselves before HIV and credited the illness with turning their lives in a positive direction.

In conclusion, the results of this tentative comparison between seropositive White gay men studied previously and Black gay men interviewed in the present study suggest that for both, HIV was a catalyst for positive change and that the search for meaning resulted, for most, in effective coping. Although no causal conclusions may be drawn concerning the effect of sociocultural influences on Black compared to White gay men, these preliminary findings suggest that the outcome of the search for meaning may be parallel even when the specific life experiences of the two groups differ significantly.

▓ Specific Sources of Meaning

Specific sources of the meaning, purpose, or value of life were explored by classifying participants' responses using the six sources identified by Schaefer and Coleman (1992) as occurring in HIV-positive White gay men's accounts of living with HIV, including relationships with others, self-discovery, acquiring knowledge, aesthetic appreciation, contributing to others, and spiritual fulfillment. As in the Schaefer and Coleman study, a thematic content analysis was used in this study to examine participants' responses. The intent in the present analysis was to determine whether similar sources of meaning would be valued by Black gay men in terms of coping with HIV.

Schaefer and Coleman (1992) reported that 17 of the 20 White gay men they interviewed said that their overall sense of meaning, purpose, and value had changed since learning of their diagnosis. For most, the change was positive. Eighteen of the men stressed that relationships with others brought the greatest sense of meaning to their lives. Partners, family members, and friends were in this category; 5 of the men also indicated that relationships with pets were significant. Ten of the men were not in a sexually committed relationship because they feared telling prospective partners they were seropositive. Self-discovery was the second most significant source of meaning to many White gay men. Awareness of their mortality led them to feel a developmental kinship to the aged. They also reported becoming less materialistic, less achievement oriented, more outer directed, or more introspective.

The three categories of acquiring knowledge, artistic expression, and contributing to others were somewhat less important to White gay men than relationships and self-discovery but still were regarded as providing an important sense of purpose (Schaefer & Coleman, 1992). Acquiring knowledge brought a sense of meaning to 15 of the White gay men. The knowledge they referred to did not concern academic learning, centering instead on information or skills that enabled them to manage HIV. Artistic appreciation and contributing to others or society both were valued by 18 participants. Artistic expression included listening to music, film making, interior design, and private reflections. Arenas for contributing to others that were meaningful included political activities, educating others about safer sex, or helping AIDS organizations. The category of meaning providing the least comfort to White gay men in

Schaefer and Coleman's study was religion or a spiritual life. A majority felt disenfranchised by mainstream religions that stigmatized homosexuality; none attended church regularly. Eight men nurtured their belief in a higher power and their spirituality through artistic expression, meditation, and visualization.

In general, the specific meanings associated with HIV obtained in the present study from interviews with seropositive Black gay men paralleled those found by Schaefer and Coleman (1992) for White gay men, with differences being observed in the path to meaning more so than in the final outcome of the search. Nearly all the participants in both groups indicated that HIV had changed their sense of the meaning of life in a positive direction. They no longer took life for granted and felt they had no time to waste. Many described taking more control of their lives by giving up addictions, eating right, exercising regularly, and focusing on what truly made them happy in their work or personal life.

In the six specific categories examined, Black gay men reported that relationships provided them with the most meaning, and spiritual fulfillment (in terms of organized religion) was seen as offering the least, similar to White gay men. The categories of acquiring knowledge, aesthetic appreciation, and contributing to others were all represented in Black gay men's accounts of finding meaning in HIV but were less important than relationships, as was also found for White gay men. However, the specific life experiences that shaped the search for meaning were different for Black gay men due to unique sociocultural influences discussed earlier, such as the effect on identity of the stigmatization of homosexuality and HIV within the Black community, as well as the consequences of coping with multiple stigmas and other sources of stress. Sociocultural influences were particularly evident for the three categories, including relationships, self-discovery, and spiritual fulfillment. In addition, the categories of acquiring knowledge, aesthetic appreciation, and contributing to others were not easily differentiated in Black gay men's accounts and were combined under the heading self-expression. Responses for each category are described below.

Relationships. The strongest sense of meaning for Black gay men living with HIV resulted from relationships with others, similar to Schaefer and Coleman (1992), although none of the Black men mentioned pets as providing a source of meaning. All Black gay men identified a significant shift in their views of relationships resulting in greater caring and commitment toward intimates, including lovers, friends, and family. However, the growth of these relationships frequently was quite difficult. Negative attitudes toward homosexuality that were perceived by participants as being widespread in the Black community were a continuing source of stress. Eleven of 13 mentioned fearing that openness about their sexual orientation would result in rejection by their families and community, effectively banishing them from their source of same-race support. They also affirmed that HIV was stigmatized as both a gay disease and a White phenomenon in their community. Cedric, age 35, explained,

> Bein' Black, if you're gay and HIV positive, you ain't worth shit! Our attitude is so bad. You'd rather be around White people than Black if you're HIV positive. . . . Many of us can't tell our families, and some are long-term survivors. Black gay men would do *anything* to keep their families. They'll stay in the closet 'til they're 90 years old! Some will take it all the way to the top of the mountain.

The expectation of rejection from this valued reference group affected 11 of the men's willingness to disclose their gay identity and HIV status to their families. (The remaining 2 men's families had become aware of their sexual orientation during their early teens; both had been thrown out of their home as a result.) Of the 11, 7 had not revealed their sexual orientation before learning they were HIV positive and were faced with the stress of coping with two concealed identities. This stress was dealt with in various ways. One told his family of his sexual orientation and HIV status simultaneously. Another, after learning 6 years ago that he was HIV positive, subsequently told his family he was gay but had not revealed his HIV status. Four told of their HIV status but did not explicitly discuss their sexual orientation, leaving their families to draw their own conclusions. Family acceptance of participants' HIV status appeared to be related to the level of acceptance of homosexuality. However, even families that had initially been rejecting of the man's homosexuality eventually responded in a supportive manner when faced with his deteriorating health.

Relations with the White community appeared to be less relevant to participants than involvement in the Black community. Eight Black gay men described the White community as quite welcoming, particularly in being more accepting of their sexual orientation and HIV status than the Black community, but most also indicated that racism prevented them from using the White community (gay or nongay) as a major and continuing source of support. Five men were unable to make comparisons because they seldom had contact with Whites.

Ten of the 13 men were not in a sexually committed relationship at the time of the interview. The burden of having to tell prospective partners of their HIV status was a strong deterrent to dating. Rejection was a common response from HIV-negative men in particular, as it was in reports from White gay men (Hoff et al., 1992). Some participants had difficulty accepting their loss of desirability, as indicated by Sebastian's (age 28) account of a recent dating experience:

> Last week I saw a guy I thought was cute. We went to my home and I told him I was HIV positive. Ten minutes later, he couldn't stand to be in the same room with me. That hurt me. No one has *ever* rejected me before. Anyone I've ever got in my clutches, I've captured with my wit and my humor and my charm. He really cracked that theology for me.

Some participants responded to rejection by reframing it in a more positive light. "Now [that I'm HIV positive] I know when someone wants to go out with me that they care about *me*, not just what they can get from me," explained Maurice (age 20).

Despite the difficulties seropositive Black gay men experienced with actual or imagined rejections, all 13 spoke of the opportunity HIV had provided for developing more intimate, meaningful relationships with family, friends, and partners, even when acceptance was slow to come. Melvin explained, "You have to have an understanding family. . . . I can go to my family now and they don't throw my cup away [after I drink from it]. They hug me and kiss me. I have people who love me." For others, the reprioritization of relationships led to important reconciliations with family members. For example, Cedric, 35 years old, described a conflicted relationship with his father that was resolved by his illness:

> HIV has given me the opportunity to have a relationship with my father I can be proud of . . . our relationship [prior to HIV] was one of long-standing hostility. He wanted me to be something he couldn't be—a professional golfer. It was a lot of pressure. . . . I went to Hawaii and many

other places just to play golf. What more could I want? But I remember conflict. . . . When I failed at some tasks, I took it out on him and me. We yelled at each other. I didn't even enjoy where I was—I was too upset. Now, ever since HIV, we've become great friends. That would be something people would say, "Cedric's life is about making peace with his father."

For two of the men, the shift resulted in allowing themselves to love and be loved for the first time. As 36-year-old Curt explained,

I'm in a relationship right now. It came completely out of the blue. I was moaning and groaning one night. "I have all these X's on my head. I'm Black. I'm gay. I'm too skinny and tall. I'm HIV positive. I'm not a marketable commodity. I will never have a special relationship." I was keeping myself at a distance. I spill all this out and the guy sitting there, out of the blue, asks me out! I felt like a school kid, I got so nervous! We're still together—we just bought a house. [What changed was that] I started taking chances for happiness.

Self-Discovery and Respect. The self-growth reported by Black gay men in the present study differed substantially in tone from that described by White gay men in Schaefer and Coleman's (1992) research. Although the Black gay men, like the Whites, became more aware of their own mortality as a result of their diagnosis, they did not spontaneously report feeling a greater kinship with the elderly or indicate being less achievement motivated, as did White men. Instead, their expressions of self-discovery had more to do with increased self-respect and a greater achievement orientation. These differences may be related to socioeconomic or age differences between the two groups. The Black gay men were substantially younger and appeared to have had fewer educational and career opportunities before HIV diagnosis than the White gay men interviewed by Schaefer and Coleman.

Catastrophic illness acted as a catalyst for 8 of the Black gay men to take more responsibility for self-improvement. Sebastian expressed this sentiment as follows:

I'm really learning that no one is obligated to love me but me. I look in the mirror. My self-image was so horrible. [I used to think] if I act really sexual, it will bring friends to me. In my pre-positive status, "Sebastian" and "sex" used to be synonymous. [But] what I am is what's *under* the body—the soul of me. I'm learning now [that] when things are going bad,

I don't need a sex partner. I'm enjoying the right to refuse. My self-esteem has increased drastically during the past year. I had people in my life that weren't worth anything. Now I have friends I can count on.

Six of the Black gay men expressed high achievement goals related to education or career or had regrets about not being able to accomplish more in those areas due to ill health. For instance, one was applying to college to study social thought and analysis, an area in which he felt his life experiences would give him a great deal to contribute. Another, Johnny Jones (age 28), spoke with great sadness about his lost opportunities:

All my life I've been a busy, busy person. I was very involved in politics. A lot of people know me as "Johnny the politician." That was my goal—to build up the trust of people and run for office. I had an internship in Washington, DC with a state senator. I've met two presidents. Since I moved here [after HIV diagnosis], I haven't established myself politically. Now I get tired. My biggest regret is that I did not go to law school. I don't think I have the stamina to do it.

Self-Expression. The three categories of acquiring knowledge, aesthetic appreciation and involvement, and contributing to others or society used by Schaefer and Coleman (1992) were combined in the present study under the heading *self-expression*. The greater valuation of the self experienced by Black gay men described above was accompanied by an intense desire to develop competencies or creative endeavors that would be beneficial to others as well as personally satisfying. For some, this meant gaining mastery over their own health care, as it did with White men in Schaefer and Coleman's research. For example, Mr. N indicated, "I've tried to be in control of my illness as much as I can. No one can take care of me like me." He was so successful at controlling his intense chronic pain due to neuropathy that a psychologist who specialized in biofeedback asked to analyze Mr. N's techniques to see if they could be used to improve his treatment of patients. This mastery was a source of pride for Mr. N.

Participants also actively sought ways to express themselves through artistic means or teaching, both of which were often aimed at contributing to others. For example, Sebastian (age 28) indicated, "I want to learn to play piano. I want to do HIV education and outreach. . . . I want to be a blessing, to administer healing. I want to open housing for transient gays. I really like the idea of sharing." Similarly, Marcus (age 31) indicated,

> I would like my future to be productive. I'm doing visiting nurse, floral work, and most of the school year [I do] HIV/AIDS education. I want a little bitty flower shop where I can create my own space. . . . [and] I'd really like a good relationship. Who wouldn't?

Lastly, those who had already contributed a great deal to their community continued to do so after becoming HIV positive. Mr. N, a cofounder of BABAA, remarked,

> One in 33 Black men are infected with HIV. If someone doesn't pick up the torch and get word out, the Black population will be crippled. Even if they don't have AIDS, they will be [HIV] positive. That won't be good for the Black or human race.

Mr. N's optimism and concern for his people sustained him as he coped with increasing medical problems.

Self-expression, including acquiring knowledge, aesthetic expression, or contributing to others, also appeared to compensate somewhat for the lack of an intimate relationship for a few participants. This was expressed very well by Maurice (age 20):

> The only thing botherin' me is not havin' a companion in my life. It's rough day by day to wake up alone. I want somebody to love in my life. That's the only thing that's missin'. . . . My life is devoted to HIV education. I didn't finish high school. I haven't seen the world, but it was never my goal. . . . I'm a support for a lot of people. I give a lot of presentations on HIV. . . . I want to get my diploma. If I could have anything [I want] it's a computer with a printer. I want to write a story about my life. I have a lot to tell . . . [but] all I've been through, it's been alone. I'm tired of fightin' by myself.

Spiritual Fulfillment. Organized religion brought the least sense of purpose to life for seropositive Black gay men, as with White gay men in Schaefer and Coleman's (1992) research, although 9 of the 13 had developed a private spirituality that sustained them. Church doctrine concerning homosexuality was one source of disenfranchisement for Black gay men, as it appeared to be for White gay men. In addition, for 10 of the 13 Black gay men, most of whom were active in their church before knowing they were seropositive, personal rejection by a minister contributed to the challenge of coping with HIV. One man explained,

> My church turned me down. I was in the church choir and word got out I was HIV positive. The pastor came to me and said, "We have to excuse you from the choir. I heard you're sick. I heard you have the package. You have to excuse yourself. We don't want your kind around our children, our choir." I said, "You tellin' me I can't come to church?" "You can come," he said, "but you have to sit in the back." I thought, "Why do I have to sit in the back?" I thought the church was supposed to be there for you to provide spiritual guidance!

However, participants responded to rejection by church leaders with creativity. Three were able to find accepting congregations after some searching, 2 in the White and 1 in the Black community. Others developed personal paths for enhancing spirituality. Still others were able to gain acceptance within the Black community by developing a new "chosen" family through their work at BABAA.

In sum, the specific outcomes of the search for meaning for Black gay men appeared to parallel those found for White gay men by Schaefer and Coleman (1992). Although the small sample size prevents firm conclusions from being drawn, sociocultural and racial influences seemed most evident for the categories of relationships, self-discovery, and spiritual fulfillment.

▨ Discussion

Several influential theories posit that the search for meaning is a basic human motivation that persists even when a person is confronted with a fate that cannot be changed, such as a diagnosis of HIV/AIDS (e.g., Antonovsky, 1987; Frankl, 1984). Under normal circumstances, meaning in life can be discovered in one of two ways: (a) by creating a work or doing a deed, or (b) experiencing something or encountering something (e.g., loving someone) (Frankl, 1984). Under unusual circumstances involving suffering, trauma, or impending death, people may not be able to aim at either of these as an ultimate goal in life. They may cease living for the future. If so, signs of hopelessness and despair may appear; the whole structure of their inner life may change. Meaning in life must then be found by realizing that when one is no longer able to change a situation, one must accept the challenge to change oneself. The attitude a person takes toward unavoidable suffering is what provides life with meaning. Thus, effective coping with trauma requires that individuals find meaning in their suffering, accept it as a unique task, and see that they may choose the way in which they bear their burden (Frankl, 1984; Yalom, 1980).

How Black gay men make sense of the trauma of living with HIV as they wait for the 7 to 10 years typically occurring between infection and illness was the focus of the present exploratory research. The results indicated that a majority of the Black gay men had achieved good psychological adaptation to HIV, similar to that reported for White gay men by Schwartzberg (1993) and Schaefer and Coleman (1992). In terms of the global meaning of HIV, most were in the categories of high and defensive meaning. These two categories represent higher levels of adaptation because the men had been able to turn their personal tragedy into an achievement by using it as an opportunity for personal growth. In contrast, those in the shattered and irrelvant meaning groups had not established meaningful life goals since their HIV diagnosis and had not adapted as well to their illness. Black gay men's high adaptation to HIV was also confirmed by comparison with Schaefer and Coleman's findings concerning the specific meanings of HIV. Each participant identified at least one positive outcome of HIV in either the area of relationships, self-respect, or self-expression.

The interpretation of findings is circumscribed by the characteristics of the specific population interviewed. All participants were self-identified as gay men. Previous research indicates that relatively few Black men who have sex with men identify themselves as homosexual; bisexual is the preferred designation of most (Peterson, 1995). However, for the HIV-positive White man who has sex with men, self-identification as a gay man is associated with greater psychological health (Leserman, DiSantostefano, Perkins, & Evans, 1994). Thus, the men included here may not be typical of the larger population of Black men who have sex with men when considering self-identification and functioning.

Sociocultural influences that appeared to have a unique impact on seropositive Black gay men's search for meaning included homophobia within the Black community, the problem of coping with dual identities and multiple stigmatizations, traumatic life histories, and rejection by important communities such as the Black church and White gay community. These preliminary findings suggest that understanding Black gay men coping with HIV cannot be done by focusing on one isolated identity or stigma. Instead, the complexity of social tasks and stressors they face must be taken into account. A potentially fruitful area of research concerns how Black gay men's search for meaning is affected by multiple identities and stigmas, including the self-protective or adaptive skills developed in response to living with prejudice.

An important treatment consideration arising from the research concerns the clinical relevance of the construct "meaning in life." Previous research has demonstrated that there is a substantial and consistent relationship between the ability to find meaning in life and psychological well-being (e.g., Debats, 1996). Thus, treatment aimed at Black gay men who have not adapted well to HIV might focus on helping them to find meaning in their experience. Religion may be a more relevant support than traditional psychotherapy for Black gay men in their search. In general, Blacks have been found to use more religious coping activities to deal with life problems than Whites and to solve problems in collaboration with God (Jackson et al., 1986). Thus one intervention that might be most clinically beneficial to Black gay men would be a compassionate response to HIV by Black religious leaders and institutions.

In conclusion, the cognitive readjustment process Black gay men underwent after learning of their seropositive status was found in the present study to involve a search for meaning. Although the search was uniquely affected by issues related to race, as well as by numerous hardships in life, most had found some meaning in their experience and confronted their illness with dignity. Those who were coping most effectively had attained a degree of inner peace and were involved actively in their community. This self-determination was a source of comfort or even joy to the men, supporting the claim of existential psychology that a sense of purpose in life helps one to grow in spite of all indignities (Frankl, 1984).

Helpful and Unhelpful Forms of Social Support for HIV-Positive Individuals

ANITA P. BARBEE
University of Louisville

VALERIAN J. DERLEGA
SUSAN P. SHERBURNE
AMY GRIMSHAW
Old Dominion University

Learning that one is HIV seropositive can create a number of stressors. The person might be concerned about dying at an early age, the pain and suffering associated with a debilitating and ultimately fatal illness, being stigmatized as an HIV or AIDS patient, or disruption in relationships with friends and family (Hays et al., 1993). One coping strategy that people use is seeking social support. There is an extensive literature on the effects of social support in coping with stressful events, but few studies have examined how the support process functions for people with

AUTHORS' NOTE: Special thanks are extended to Jennifer Baddgett, Jenny Caja, Kevin Reichmuth, Crescent Smith, and Pamela Thompson for transcribing the interviews. Our gratitude is also extended to the individuals who talked with us about their personal experiences living with the HIV infection, which provided the material for this chapter.

HIV or AIDS (Hays, Catania, McKusick, & Coates, 1990; Hays et al., 1992). This chapter has three purposes: (a) to review briefly the literature on social support for HIV/AIDS patients, (b) to focus on a model that we developed to study the social support process in close relationships (Barbee & Cunningham, 1995), and (c) to present in-depth personal account data from a study designed to examine supportive interactions involving HIV-seropositive individuals as participants.

Literature on Social Support for HIV-Positive Individuals

Several studies have examined whether being diagnosed as HIV positive or having AIDS is associated with more support seeking. Hays, Catania, et al. (1990) found that gay men who were diagnosed as either HIV positive or as having AIDS sought help more than gay men who were HIV negative or who were unaware of their HIV status. Additionally, those diagnosed with HIV who used active forms of coping such as coming up with strategies about what to do and seeing the problem in a more positive light sought support more than those who were in denial or who used other avoidant forms of coping such as acting as if the situation were hopeless (Leserman, Perkins, & Evans, 1992). Black gay men in that study were more likely to use denial as a coping strategy and to receive less social support from their network members.

Other studies have examined to whom HIV-positive individuals turn after the diagnosis. All of the studies found that friends were the most frequently sought sources of support by gay men who are HIV positive (Catania, Turner, Choi, & Coates, 1992; Hays, Catania, et al., 1990; Hays, Chauncey, & Tobey, 1990). Lovers are also important sources of support (Hays, Chauncey, & Tobey, 1990). Only about a third of the time did people with AIDS turn to family members; even then, siblings were prefered to parents (Hays, Chauncey, & Tobey, 1990). Hays et al. (1993) reported that friends and lovers provided more help to gay men with HIV infection than did relatives and colleagues. In a follow-up study, Hays et al. (1993) found that support from friends and lovers at Time 1 was correlated with less depression and anxiety 1 year later at Time 2. They also found that the more help gay men with AIDS received from their mothers, the more psychological distress they experienced. However, Catania et al. found that perceived positive support from family was more strongly related to less death anxiety than that received from peers. Thus, it is reasonable for gay men suffering with AIDS to turn most often to friends and lovers, especially in the early stages of the disease, but making peace with family members as health problems increase or as death approaches may help people with AIDS cope more effectively (Yankeelov, 1995).

Finally, studies have examined the effect of social support on mental and physical well-being among persons with HIV or AIDS. Hays, Chauncey, and Tobey (1990) found that the fewer close associates gay men with AIDS had, the more depression they experienced. The greater the proportion of friends in their overall network, the happier they were, and the greater the proportion of gay friends in their network, the less anxious they were. Leserman et al. (1992) found that people who coped in a proactive fashion not only received more support but were more satisfied with the support they received and felt less depressed than those who were in denial about the illness. Likewise, Kelly and his colleagues (1993) found that HIV-positive individuals with high perceived social support had lower depression scores.

Certain types of support have been associated with particular outcomes as well. For instance, emotional and informational support were most predictive of overall well-being in the Hays, Chauncey, and Tobey (1990) study. These forms of support, plus tangible support, were associated with less depression in the Hays et al. (1992) study. Furthermore, Hays et al. (1992) found that satisfaction with informational support was especially critical in buffering the stress associated with HIV symptoms. One study examined support given in the asymptomatic versus symptomatic stages of the disease (Pakenham, Dadds, & Terry, 1994). This research found that in the asymptomatic stage of the illness, emotional support was associated with a better subjective health status and better social adjustment. However, having a romantic partner was associated with poorer social adjustment and an increased number of symptoms for the symptomatic group. The conclusion from these findings was that overprotectiveness was very unhelpful in symptomatic AIDS patients.

In summary, then, gay men who are diagnosed as either HIV positive or as having AIDS symptoms are much like others suffering from a life-threatening illness (e.g., Lehman, Ellard, & Wortman, 1986). They seek support more than those who have not been diagnosed with the illness. They seek it most from close associates, and they benefit the most from emotional, informational, and tangible aid. These forms of support are associated with less depression and anxiety and greater psychological and physical well-being. The main difference in this group from patients with other illnesses is that the support network configuration is slightly different. Gay men turn to friends the most, lovers second, and family last when seeking aid in coping with their diagnosis. Studies of people coping with cancer, death, and other ailments have found spouses and family tops on the list of sources of social support (Dakof & Taylor, 1990; Lehman et al., 1986). This difference is probably due to the way that gay men have structured their lives previous to the diagnosis. Because of their sexual orientation, many gay men are estranged from disapproving family members; thus friends and lovers in the gay community become "family."

There are several limitations to the research on support for people who are HIV positive. Thus far, the emphasis has been on white, middle class, gay males who are diagnosed as either HIV positive or as having AIDS (Hays, Catania, et al., 1990; Hays, Chauncey, & Tobey, 1990; Hays et al., 1992; Pakenham et al., 1994; Siegel & Krauss, 1991). Of the studies we found, only two examined reactions of black gay men (Kelly et al., 1993; Leserman et al., 1992) and only one included a sample of women, but even this one had only 15 women in a total sample of 142 (Kelly et al., 1993). Thus, more research is needed on those diagnosed with AIDS who are people of color, from the lower classes, heterosexual, and female. For example, we may find that family members are sought for support more often among people of color, heterosexuals, and women than among white gay males.

Now that studies have established that support is associated with less psychological distress in HIV/AIDS patients, more research is needed that examines the specific behaviors enacted toward individuals with HIV, the nature of those behaviors in terms of being helpful or unhelpful, how those behaviors are perceived by individuals with HIV, and how those behaviors are related to well-being. To move the research in this direction, a brief description of our approach to the study of social support is necessary.

Sensitive Interaction Systems Theory

To clarify the relation between help-seeking behaviors, social support behaviors, and various positive and negative outcomes, Barbee and her colleagues (Barbee et al., 1993; Barbee & Cunningham, 1995) developed Sensitive Interaction Systems Theory (SIST). A central postulate of SIST is that distressed individuals have a general sense of the form of support that they want, and partners usually wish to be supportive, but a host of internal and external variables can produce conflicting motives, tension, or ambiguity in the process of asking for or providing social support. Mixed messages and misperceptions in the communication process can, in turn, cause social support interactions to be less than helpful. This may be particularly true of HIV-positive individuals during a support interaction.

Several factors could influence an HIV-positive individual's willingness to ask clearly for help. The HIV individual's own feelings about the disease and how he or she acquired it, his or her feelings about the person from whom help is needed, and the type of help that is needed could all influence whether and how he or she asks for support. Some of the same factors could also influence the willingness and ability of a potential helper to give support (Barbee, 1990).

In many cases, the support that is given is helpful and leads to positive outcomes for the recipient. Unfortunately, interacting with members of one's support network does not always have these positive emotional and physical effects. There have been studies that found that interacting with members of one's network when under stress can produce a decrease in well-being (Rook, 1984). Coworkers may say something that is perceived as unhelpful, such as "What happened to you is God's will" (e.g., Lehman et al., 1986). Family may behave in a manner that implicitly stigmatizes. Parents, for example, might require their son who has AIDS to eat from paper plates when he visits for Thanksgiving dinner.

In some cases in which social support is disappointing, the social support seeker may have failed to employ effective behaviors to elicit support from the friend (Gulley, 1993). In other cases of social support failure, the friend may have been unwilling or unable to provide the form of support that was needed by the help seeker to handle the specific type of stressful problem.

SIST notes that sources of ambivalence within the helper may influence the type of behavior (from among several specified by the interactive coping typology) that the helper provides. *Approach* behaviors include both problem-focused *solve* behaviors to find the answer to the problem, such as making suggestions, and emotion-focused *solace* behaviors to elicit positive emotion in the seeker and express closeness, such as complimenting the friend. *Avoidance* behaviors include both problem-focused *dismiss* behaviors to minimize the significance of the problem, such as saying the problem is not serious, and emotion-focused *escape* behaviors to discourage the display of negative emotion or to distract the person, such as making fun of the person's distress.

The research that has distinguished between helpful and unhelpful forms of support towards HIV-positive individuals has focused on *who* is more likely to give *positive* forms of support, rather than detailing the form in which these types of support manifest themselves and the reasons they are given.

Our past research found that most recipients prefer solve and solace behaviors over dismiss and escape behaviors for minor problems (Barbee, 1990). It is not clear that the same preferences exist with major problems. Studies of people coping with cancer or the death of a loved one found that some forms of solve behaviors, like giving advice, were not welcomed (e.g., Lehman et al., 1986).

We conducted a study that sought to understand how HIV-positive individuals view the support that they are given, using our typology of interactive social support. We predicted that more of our sample (which has diversity in terms of gender, sexual orientation, cause of infection, and education level) would rely on family than in the gay male samples of past studies. We also predicted that the approach behaviors of solve and solace would be most representative of the helpful behaviors and that escape and dismiss behaviors would be most representative of the unhelpful behaviors.

▨ Method

Research Participants

Forty-two people with a mean age of 34 who were either HIV positive (62%) or who also had AIDS (38%) were recruited from HIV/AIDS community support groups in southeastern Virginia. Our sample was similar to those in other studies that focus on HIV and social support because other studies and our own included primarily homosexual males who contracted the disease through sexual contact. Our sample differed from other samples in that most of our participants had grown up and remained in Virginia. Most of our research participants were African

American (68%), less educated (only 38% had either attended college or received a college degree), unemployed (86%), and living in poverty (71% made less than $10,000 a year). We also had 14% women in the sample, 21% heterosexuals, and 14% who contracted the disease from behaviors other than sexuality. Most other studies sample HIV-positive persons who tend to be white, middle-class professionals. Thus the diversity of our sample may give us important information about the support process as it unfolds among individuals with HIV or AIDS who are not usually participants in research.

In our sample, 31% had a mother who was deceased and 43% had a father who was deceased. Thus, a large number had already lost a major potential source of support. Eighty-eight percent, however, felt that they had someone they could talk to about the disease. Many respondents (55%) reported talking to a friend, 21% said they talk to a romantic partner, another 21% reported talking to a family member, and very few (3%) reported talking to a coworker about being HIV positive.

We did not include health professionals as an option in the question about whether the person had someone special with whom to talk about having the HIV infection. But when we examined the personal accounts generated by the participants concerning support episodes, 86% reported a helpful or unhelpful interaction with a health professional. Furthermore, 83% reported an interaction with a friend, 83% reported an interaction with a family member, 33% reported an interaction with a romantic partner, 29% mentioned an interaction with a coworker, and 12% reported interactions with clergy. A surprising 31% mentioned interactions with a stranger in their accounts.

Many participants in our study had concerns about their health. The average CD4 cell count was 290.8. Over half of the sample was experiencing shortness of breath, a cough, a rash, fatigue, weight loss, and swollen glands. Forty-nine percent reported fair to poor health. Thus, the implications of the illness were salient for many of the research participants at the time of the interviews.

Interview Procedure

Participants in the study were interviewed in private offices at an HIV/AIDS counseling organization for a period of 45 to 90 min. The focus of the interview was on the individual's experiences with social support provided by others, as well as the reasons for disclosing or not disclosing HIV seropositive test results to others (see Chapter 8).

Each participant was asked a series of questions about instances when someone thought they were being "supportive" but whose behavior was actually "helpful" or "not helpful" in coping with the HIV infection. Each interview was audiotaped and subsequently transcribed. After the transcripts were made, two additional students coded the tapes for helpful and unhelpful acts.

Coding of the Transcripts

First, all support behaviors were unitized. Each unit consisted of one sentence. Once all 435 unitized acts were written out, each was labeled as either helpful or unhelpful according to the characterization by the research participant. Then two coders rated each behavior according to the Barbee Interactive Coping Behavior Coding System (ICBCS) (Barbee, 1990; Barbee & Cunningham, 1995). Behaviors were rated as belonging to one of four categories: solve, solace, dismiss, or escape. *Solve* behaviors include asking questions about the details of the problem, trying to figure out the cause of the problem, giving suggestions on how to solve the problem, giving information to help the person solve the problem, and doing something active or physical to help the needy person. *Solace* behaviors included giving affection, showing understanding and empathy, complimenting the needy person, assuring the person of future availability to help, reassuring the person, doing things to try to lift their mood such as buying them gifts, and asking them how they feel about the problem. *Dismiss* behaviors were changing the topic of conversation, showing disinterest in the problem, criticizing the way the person handles the problem, minimizing the severity of the problem, ridiculing the person about the problem, and feigning sympathy with pollyannaish statements. *Escape* behaviors involved refusing to speak to the other person, trying to distract the person, escaping nonverbally by refusing to listen, encouraging the needy person to escape and have fun, making fun of the person's reaction to the problem, showing irritation with the person, saying mean things to the person, and encouraging the person to suppress their negative emotions. The Cohen's kappa was .93.

Thus the transcripts were coded for who gave the support (friends, lovers, family members, health professionals, coworkers, clergy, or strang-

TABLE 5.1   Types of Social Support Provided by Various Individuals (in percentages)

	Lovers	Friends	Family	Health Professionals
Solve	18	31	32	41
Solace	38	41	29	31
Dismiss	18	5	12	15
Escape	25	22	27	14
Total	100	100	100	100

NOTE: These data were collapsed across helpful and unhelpful acts.

ers), the evaluation of the support that was given (helpful or unhelpful), and the category of the support (solve, solace, dismiss, or escape).

▧ Results

Who Gave Support

Participants generated a total number of 435 helpful and unhelpful acts across 256 supportive episodes. All of the data reported in this section refer to the *acts* rather than the *episodes*, which could have several acts within them. Thirty-five percent were acts from lovers and friends, 26% were from family members, 27% were from health care professionals, 10% were from coworkers and strangers, and 2% were from clergy or God. Thus 63% of the supportive acts were from close associates and 37% were from less close associates.

Who Gave What Types of Support

When looking at the total number of potentially supportive acts, about one-third were from lovers and friends combined and the other two-thirds were fairly equally distributed among family members and health care professionals. In further breaking those down into "helpful" and "unhelpful" forms of support, we found out why participants preferred friends to others in seeking support. Sixty-two percent of stories about friends were about acts that were helpful; only 38% of stories about friends were about acts that were unhelpful. This may partially be due to the fact that the most frequent behavior from friends across all types of support was to give solace (see Table 5.1).

TABLE 5.2   Mean Number of Types of Social Support Acts

Variable	Mean	Standard Deviation	Percentage
Number of total support acts	10.34	4.96	100
Number of helpful acts	5.71	3.47	55
Number of unhelpful acts	4.64	2.79	45
Breakdown of helpful and unhelpful acts			
Number of solves	3.38	2.79	33
Number of solaces	3.50	2.32	34
Number of dismisses	1.07	1.44	10
Number of escapes	2.41	1.91	23

Interestingly, a similar pattern was found for health care professionals in that 67% of the acts reported about health care professionals were about them being helpful and only 33% of the acts reported were about them being unhelpful. Health professionals were most likely to be remembered giving solve behaviors, which fits their role (see Table 5.1).

The pattern for lovers and family members was quite different, however. Half of the acts in the interactions with lovers were positive, but the other half were negative. A majority (62%) of interactions with family members were about unhelpful actions whereas only 38% of interactions with family members were about helpful actions.

Types of Support

As expected, participants reported slightly more helpful acts. Fifty-five percent of the reported acts were rated as helpful, but 45% were rated as unhelpful. Thirty-three percent of the behaviors were categorized as solve behaviors and 34% were categorized as solace, for a total of 67% "approach" support behaviors. Remember that solve and solace behaviors are both types of support that help the recipient approach or deal directly with their problem or the emotions it produces, whereas escape and dismiss behaviors are both types of support that lead the recipient to avoid their problems or the emotional aftermath. Twenty-three percent of the behaviors were categorized as escape behaviors, but only 10% of the behaviors were categorized as dismiss, for a total of 33% "avoidant" behaviors (see Table 5.2).

TABLE 5.3   Percentages of Types of Helpful and Unhelpful
            Support Acts

	Helpful	*Unhelpful*
Solve	42	23
Solace	53	7
Dismiss	3	19
Escape	2	51

Helpful Forms of Support

The interviewer asked each participant what people in their network did that was helpful and what was done that was unhelpful. This type of data enables us to understand how the HIV positive participants viewed the various helpful and unhelpful behaviors. First, we looked at the frequency of each type of specific behavior described as helpful and compared that information to our interactive coping typology (Barbee & Cunningham, 1995). An overwhelming majority of those behaviors that were rated as helpful were in the solve (42%) and solace (53%) categories (see Table 5.3).

Most of the solve behaviors were in the form of "tangible aid" (60%) such as giving money, food, medications, clothing, transportation, and helping with expenses, chores, care of children, self-care, navigating the system, joining support groups, and moving. Another 18% of solve behaviors involved "giving suggestions for how to solve the problem" or suggestions on resources to help with the problem such as getting further testing, getting more information about the disease, seeing a psychiatrist, and suggestions on how to avoid depression and how to eat and sleep properly. Eleven percent of the solves involved "asking questions about the problem" such as how the person was coping with the news, how the disease was contracted, how the asker could help, and what the person's future plans would be. The final types of solve behaviors (12%) involved "helping the person to understand the cause of the disease" and expressing hope that research and new medications promise reduced symptoms or a possible end to the threat of death.

The solace behaviors included all of the behaviors we include in our theoretically based coding system (Barbee & Cunningham, 1995). The most prominent included "availability" (33%) such as promising to be there for the HIV-positive person, taking off work to spend time with the HIV-positive person, and talking with the person about his or her feelings. "Affection" was also frequently mentioned (17%) in the form of the willingness of close others to give hugs, kisses, and touches as well as to put their arm around the HIV-positive person, declare their love for the HIV person, and indicate a willingness to have sex with the HIV person. A great deal of "mood lifting" (18%) occurred, such as telling jokes, giving cards, giving gifts, being really up, taking a walk with the HIV-positive person, taking the person out to dinner or lunch, getting the HIV-positive person involved in volunteer work, taking the person to the symphony, baking a cake for the person, and swapping recipes with the person. Another 18% of the behaviors were in the form of "reassurance," including saying the life of the HIV-positive person was not over, that the person would be able to figure out how to cope, defending the person, and saying everything would be OK. Seven percent of helpers "asked about how the person was feeling." Another 4% "gave compliments" to the person, including asking the HIV-infected person to organize an AIDS ministry for their church, asking them to give speeches, seeing them as an inspiration, asking them to sing in their wedding, and saying things such as "you have such a positive and bright attitude about everything" and "they would come and tell stories about me and how I had influenced their lives." Two percent of the behaviors involved "empathy," including crying with the HIV-positive person, being understanding of the behavior that led to AIDS, and showing their own feelings of upset. Finally, only 1% of the behaviors included "promises of privacy and confidentiality" about the shared information of the person's HIV status.

Three percent of the helpful forms of support were from the dismiss category and 2% were escape behaviors. The helpful dismiss behaviors primarily tried to minimize the seriousness of the disease. Examples included, "you could live 20-30 years, you never know" or "even though you have HIV, you are still alive." Other helpful dismiss statements tried to keep the participant from thinking about the problem such as "don't really think about it" or "don't put so much into it." Still others were said with humor such as "well, we all have to go sometime" and "he told me I was HIV positive in a comical way."

The helpful escape behaviors sometimes tried to distract the person from the weight of the devastating emotions. For instance, "he made me keep working and keep my mind occupied so that I wouldn't keep thinking about it." Other examples encouraged the patient to escape and have fun to forget about it all, such as saying "regardless, we are still here . . . let's go out and party."

Although dismiss and escape behaviors were occasionally seen as helpful, the results were similar to our findings in previous research on people's perceptions of support for everyday problems. Approach behaviors were seen more positively than avoidance behaviors. When avoidance behaviors were seen as helpful, skill was evident in minimizing the HIV person's anxiety through the use of distraction and playing down the severity of the problem.

Unhelpful Forms of Support

After examining the helpful behaviors, we looked at the unhelpful behaviors in a similar way. Unlike the categorization of helpful acts, 51% of the unhelpful acts were escape behaviors and 19% were dismiss behaviors, thus 70% of the unhelpful behaviors were avoidant in nature.

Our findings in this study were somewhat different from our previous research, which focused on people coping with everyday problems rather than major life events or life-threatening illnesses. However, the results were more similar to the findings of Dakof and Taylor (1990) and Lehman et al. (1986), who did study people facing illness and coping with death. We found that 23% of the unhelpful behaviors were in the solve category and 7% were in the solace category. Thus, nearly one-third of the unhelpful acts were from the behaviors that are often seen as positive. The unwanted solve behaviors were from many of the usual categories of solve but may have been interpreted as being an invasion of privacy or as an attempt to take control of the patient or the situation. Many unwanted solves involved a loved one asking too many personal questions about how the disease was contracted, how long the patient had had the disease, and, as in the case of one father, "he pumped me for health information that I wasn't ready to give." Many unwanted solves were forms of advice, such as "she said get tested again," "he tried to tell me what was good for me," or "you'd better put yourself in a home because you never know when you might fall sick." Many other unhelpful solves were instances of offering tangible assistance, such as offering for the patient to move in with them, offering to pay bills, or offers of general assistance such as "she tried to take over," "they wanted me to sign over power of attorney to them," and "she overcompensated and helped too much." Still other unhelpful solves were instances of giving facts about the disease and its treatment, for instance, "It's a life or death situation, if you don't take the medication you're gonna die" or misinformation, for instance, "my friend's information about HIV was very off the wall."

The unwanted solace behaviors came in several forms. Often the person was trying to lift the mood of the patient by sending cards, by taking them to dinner, or by giving gifts to the patient. However, many of these behaviors were recounted with commentary like "she bought me a gift out of pity" or "everyone sent Xmas cards that they normally don't." Others felt smothered with availability such as "she calls me *every day*" or "she kept giving me all this attention." Still others hated receiving affection as in this case, "she *always* put her arm around me and asked me how I was doing." Still other helpers were trying to show empathy by being sad "with" the patient or by showing their own anxiety about the patient's illness. For instance, "he cries and just can't accept the fact that one day I'm not going to be here."

We found several distinguishing aspects of those solve and solace behaviors that were seen as helpful and those that were seen as unhelpful. For example, when asking questions, a helper's behavior was seen as more negative when the HIV person could detect insincerity or when the question was personally intrusive. In the case of perspective taking, helpful people reframed the situation in a positive light without mentioning the negatives, but unhelpful people reframed in such a way as to remind the HIV person of their mortality. Helpful suggestions were given in a tentative fashion, whereas unhelpful suggestions showed overprotectiveness and were often in the form of orders. In the same way, tangible aid that was unhelpful was enacted in a more overt and overbearing fashion than helpful offers of tangible assistance. For example, one helpful mother slipped some money to the HIV daughter, whereas another mother took over the daughter's life by paying all of her bills for her. Overall, the unhelpful solves were more intrusive and showed clear signs of the helper's anxiety.

Similarly, the unwanted solaces bordered on irritating because they were overdone. Phrases like "kept giving," "can't accept the fact," "normally don't," and "out of pity" came up continually when describing the unhelpful solace behaviors. There was also the sense that people who were unhelpful were insincere and that they were giving support conditionally. These kinds of phrases and feelings of irritation did not emerge in the wanted solace descriptions.

The Relationship Between Age and Health Status With Social Support

To examine the effects of various demographic variables on the expression of social support, we correlated age, number of siblings, and CD4 cell count with number of helpful and unhelpful support acts from lovers, friends, families, and health professionals as well as the number of acts that were coded as solves, solaces, dismisses, and escapes.

We found that older participants were less likely to report about support behaviors from romantic partners ($r = -.31$) and slightly more likely to report about support behaviors from health professionals ($r = .27$). When a person had more siblings, there was a trend for reporting on fewer support behaviors from friends ($r = -.26$).

In terms of the relationships with health status, the higher the CD4 cell count, the greater the number of supportive solace acts participants reported receiving ($r = .33$), with slightly more dismiss behaviors as well ($r = .26$). When the CD4 cell count was higher, there was also a trend for recounting more support behaviors from health professionals ($r = .27$). Higher CD4 cell counts mean that a person is healthier, thus the findings suggest that the healthier an HIV-positive individual is, the more support they receive, especially from health professionals, although some of it is dismissive. No other correlations were significant (see Table 5.4 for correlation matrix).

Effects of Race, Gender, Sexual Orientation, Cause of HIV Infection, and Job Status on Social Support

Because our sample was more diverse than other samples studying social support among HIV-positive individuals, we wanted to explore the effects of various demographic categories on the receipt of helpful and unhelpful forms of support. Thus we conducted separate analyses of variance using race, gender, sexual orientation, how HIV was contracted, and job status as independent variables. The dependent variables examined were amount of helpful and unhelpful acts; number of solves, solaces, dismisses, and escapes received; and number of acts from family

TABLE 5.4 Correlations Among Solve, Solace, Dismiss, Escape, and Other Variables (N = 42)

	Age	Number of Siblings	CD4 Cell Count	Lover	Friend	Family	Health Professional	Solve	Solace	Dismiss	Escape
Age	1.00										
Number of Siblings	.03	1.00									
CD4 Cell Count	.07	.06	1.00								
Number of supportive behaviors provided by:											
Lover	-.31**	.06	.17	1.00							
Friend	.05	-.26*	.14	-.06	1.00						
Family	-.21	.09	-.21	-.01	.10	1.00					
Health professional	.27*	.14	.27*	-.17	-.19	-.09	1.00				
Number of behaviors in the category of:											
Solve	.04	-.15	-.10	-.15	.33**	.42***	.30**	1.00			
Solace	-.07	-.05	.33**	.17	.54***	.28*	.09	.05	1.00		
Dismiss	.07	-.15	.26*	.15	.09	.17	.31**	.17	.41**	1.00	
Escape	-.13	.05	.10	.19	.32**	.43***	.04	.12	.62***	.06	1.00

*$p < .10$; **$p < .05$; ***$p < .01$.

members, friends, romantic partners, health professionals, and others. There were no significant effects for sexual orientation on receipt of any type of support or support provider.

How a person became HIV positive produced several effects. People who contracted the HIV infection from a blood transfusion ($M = 7.00$) were more likely to report receiving solve behaviors, $F(2, 35) = 3.26$, $p < .05$, than did those who received the disease from unprotected sex or from intravenous drug use. Those who received HIV from unprotected sex ($M = 3.34$) received more solve behaviors than those who received it from intravenous drug use ($M = 1.67$).

Those who contracted HIV from intravenous drug use ($M = 2.33$) were more likely to recount incidents of helpful and unhelpful acts of social support from romantic partners than those who contracted HIV from either unprotected sex ($M = 0.53$) or from a blood transfusion ($M = 0.33$), $F(2, 35) = 3.92, p < .03$.

White participants ($M = 5.80$) recounted slightly more unhelpful behaviors than did black participants ($M = 4.21$), $F(1, 36) = 3.20, p < .08$. Additionally, white participants ($M = 4.30$) reported overall more supportive interactions with family members than did black participants ($M = 2.04$), $F(1, 36) = 11.42, p < .002$. We found a high positive correlation between number of unhelpful behaviors and number of interactions with family members for white participants ($r = .51$, but for black participants $r = .32$, *ns*). Thus one reason why whites reported more unwanted acts may be because they reported more acts from family members than did blacks.

When examining the effect of gender, we found that females reported more overall support, $F(1, 37) = 8.66, p < .006$; more solves, $F(1, 37) = 4.44, p < .04$; more solaces, $F(1, 37) = 3.90, p < .05$; and more overall support from romantic partners, $F(1, 37) = 3.37, p < .07$, than did males.

Those who were employed reported more dismiss behaviors, $F(1, 40) = 8.11, p < .007$, than those who were not employed.

Discussion

We found that most of our HIV-positive sample had someone with whom they could talk about their disease. When they were asked to list those to whom they talk for support, just as in previous research on support among AIDS patients (e.g., Hays, Catania, et al. 1990), about half reported talking to friends about their HIV- or AIDS-related problems. About one fifth listed lovers as confidants, and another fifth listed a family member as a source of support.

When we asked our research participants to give personal accounts of helpful and unhelpful situations, however, most of the participants had a story about how a health professional treated them, and an equal number of the participants reported a story about a friend or a family member. Only one third recounted a story about a lover, and, as expected, only about one third reported a conversation with a coworker or a stranger. Thus, even though they frequently received support from a friend concerning their problems, participants often had support encounters with health professionals and family members. We did not ask the participants if they were currently in a romantic relationship, thus the lower occurrence of those types of interactions may be an artifact of not currently having that type of relationship. Most people have friends, and some have contact with a part of their family but may not be involved with anyone romantically. However, it may be the case that even though fewer interactions occur with romantic partners, the few interactions HIV-positive people do have are salient and powerful in their impact because of the close nature of the relationship.

We found out that participants preferred friends to others in seeking support (on the basis of their answer to the question about having someone special with whom to talk about their HIV status), probably because friends were more likely to be helpful and particularly likely to give solace when support was sought. Lovers and family members were often seen as unhelpful.

Thus our overall pattern of results confirms past research that finds friends as preferred confidants for HIV-positive persons. There are two important aspects of this finding. First, our results replicate findings that used samples of primarily urban, middle-class, white, homosexual populations. The fact that we interviewed both black and white, male and female HIV-positive individuals who were largely low income and from a smaller metropolitan area expands the external validity of previous work. Our study also gives us some insight as to why friends are preferred confidants. Although a great number of support interactions that the HIV-positive individuals are having are with health professionals and family members as well as friends, the support interactions they recall with family members tend to be simply less pleasant and helpful than the ones with friends (Hays et al., 1993).

Types of Support Recalled and How the Support Was Received

As expected, we found that most of the helpful behaviors were from the solve and solace category; very few were from the dismiss and escape categories. This confirms our belief that the best way to give support is by offering solace and giving informational support and tangible aid. Sometimes minimizing the problem and helping the person escape is helpful, but not often, even for uncontrollable problems. Most of the dismiss and escape behaviors were seen as unhelpful.

We found that it was not enough to know the percentage of each type of support, because the same acts of support might be labeled as helpful or not helpful based on the social context in which the behavior occurred. Thus, the perceptions of the recipients are important in determining the meaningfulness and helpfulness of particular behaviors. In this study, for example, about a third of the unhelpful behaviors were from the "positive" solve and solace categories. The same behaviors that many participants found to be helpful were precisely the behaviors that other participants found to be unhelpful.

We can interpret these findings in several ways. When a problem is largely out of a person's control, influences every aspect of his or her life, and is long term, giving advice may be seen as either critical or insensitive. The person needing the help knows that little can be done to change the outcome of the situation, so proposed solutions, especially if they are unsolicited, may be irritating.

Our participants also saw the unwanted solace behaviors as often stemming from undesired pity, which demeaned their dignity. Excessive expressions of concern, such as calling every day to ask how the person is feeling, could convey that the person is seen as helpless.

These findings are very important in juxtaposition with the findings that emotional, informational, and tangible support were predictive of well-being in other studies (Hays, Catania, et al., 1990; Hays et al., 1992). Although most of the time support in the form of information, tangible aid, and solace is welcomed and leads to well-being, sometimes it does not. About one third of the time, the HIV-positive individuals in our interview sample did not welcome such "positive" forms of support. When these types of support were unwelcome, they caused our participants to feel worse after the interaction rather than better.

Reasons That a Helper Fails to Be Helpful

It is probably the case that family members are well meaning in trying to offer advice, tangible aid, and solace to their child or sibling who is dying. Our work on SIST (Barbee & Cunningham, 1995) reminds us that family members may be trying to cope with the tragedy of losing a loved one to AIDS at the same time they are trying to give effective forms of support to the person living with HIV and/or AIDS. Sometimes family members' attempts to take over the care of their relative is an attempt to make *themselves* feel more in control of the situation, as a form of active coping with the thought that their family member may die. This type of help may appear intrusive to the ill relative. Other times, family members may feel that the sick person really wants this type of help. In either case, family members may not be aware of how their behaviors are coming across because they are so inwardly focused on managing their own negative emotions around the situation. Their insensitivity may be harmful to the AIDS patient, but it is also understandable given their own coping needs (Greif & Porembski, 1988).

Further support for the notion that family members may be coping with serious negative emotions themselves is reflected in the fact that of the escape behaviors recalled in the sample, the majority, 30%, were enacted by family members. Thus, family members may use escape behaviors to avoid dealing with their own feelings of distress about the HIV-seropositive status of their relative.

In further examination of the data on who was most likely to give different types of support, we found that health professionals were more likely than others to give problem-focused solve and dismiss behaviors, whereas friends and family were more likely than others to give emotion-focused solace and escape behaviors. This finding is consistent with the different roles that each plays in the life of the HIV-positive person. The health professional is trained to focus on the problem itself and how to either solve it or minimize it in the life of the patient. Close associates, on the other hand, are more emotionally involved with the patient and thus are more likely than others to engage in emotion-focused support giving.

Implications for Family and Friends

Health professionals, family members, lovers, and friends of individuals with HIV and AIDS need to be aware that advice, tangible assistance, and emotional support will not always be seen as helpful or desirable. We would recommend that, to insure that the power to decide will reside with the HIV-seropositive person, these close associates ask individuals with HIV and AIDS what they want and how they want to be treated rather than assuming that advice or help will be welcomed. This will give the HIV-seropositive person yet another way to feel in control over his or her life.

Thus far we can conclude, given the relatively high rate at which escape, dismiss, and some types of solve behaviors were seen as unwanted, that those who seek to be supportive of those who are HIV positive may be advised to emphasize solace behaviors. The best approach, however, may be to establish clear communications with the HIV-positive person about what form of support is desired at what times. By understanding the dynamics of the social support process and how HIV-positive individuals view the help that they receive, we can assist those who love them to better give the support that they truly need.

We recommend that health professionals and caretakers receive training on how to cope with the news that their patient or close associate has been diagnosed with a deadly disease. Training could also include strategies for supporting the person with HIV/AIDS, with clear information about how to behave so as not to offend the person.

Implications for Individuals With the HIV Infection

People with HIV need to understand the grief that their family members are going through and why their grief makes them overbearing and controlling. Paradoxically, someone with the HIV infection may also need to be supportive of grieving family members and be understanding and forgiving when they sometimes act insensitively. The news about being HIV seropositive may be devastating not only for the person diagnosed with HIV; it may also consitute a tragedy for family members and close friends. Mutual and interactive coping (in the form of both giving and receiving social support) needs to be engaged in by both family members and the person with the HIV infection.

Implications for Future Research

Although our sample was diverse, our small sample size was able to unearth only a few differences due to gender or race. As is usually found in the social support literature (Barbee et al., 1993), women reported overall more support acts and received more of the positive forms of help, solves and solaces. Women also reported more support from lovers than did men. This finding was complicated by the fact that all of the women in the sample were heterosexual and most of the men were homosexual. Thus we are not certain whether the additional help for women by romantic partners was a function of their gender or their sexual orientation. Future research needs to explore the ease of providing social support in various types of male and female relationships (homosexual versus heterosexual). These findings do, however, extend our knowledge of how support functions for women who are HIV positive.

In terms of race, our results for white people with the HIV infection mirrors findings with other white subjects in that their interactions with family members included both supportive and nonsupportive behaviors. Our data does suggest that blacks who are HIV positive may receive fewer unwanted support behaviors than whites who are ill with the virus (see Chapter 4). However, more comparative research with larger samples needs to be conducted to examine these and other differences in the experiences of white and black victims of the disease.

Finally, how a person contracts HIV influences the type of support they remember receiving. People who contracted HIV through means that are commonly viewed as out of their control (e.g., from a blood transfusion) were more likely to report receiving solve behaviors than those who received the disease from more controllable causes such as unprotected sex or illegal drug use. Drug users received the least amount of solve behaviors than any other group but received more from lovers than did others. It may be the case that the lovers of these participants were also drug users and thus were less judgmental of the ill person's state. Again, more research is needed to examine the effects of cause of disease on social interactions.

▓ Conclusions

This chapter shows how individuals with the HIV infection may be the recipients of social support that is perceived as helpful or unhelpful. Although HIV-positive individuals may have a clear sense of what kinds of supportive interactions are helpful, support providers (e.g., family, lovers, friends, and health professionals) and support recipients may sometimes experience conflicting motives, tensions, and misperceptions that can get in the way of these helpful behaviors being enacted and appreciated.

Helping in Hard Times
Relationship Closeness and the
AIDS Volunteer Experience

ALLEN M. OMOTO
DIANA ODOM GUNN
A. LAUREN CRAIN
University of Kansas

Responses to the global HIV epidemic have ranged broadly. International health organizations have collected epidemiological data, the U.S. Congress has debated over funding for AIDS programs, and pharmaceutical companies have developed new drugs and new uses for existing drugs to combat HIV disease. At the level of the individual, people have made and continue to make decisions about whether or not they will engage in behaviors that put them at risk for HIV and whether or not they will take responsibility for helping fight HIV in their commu-

AUTHORS' NOTE: The research reported here and preparation of this chapter were supported by research grants from the National Institute of Mental Health. The authors thank the staff and volunteers at the Columbus AIDS Task Force, Columbus, OH, the Good Samaritan Project, Kansas City, MO, and the Minnesota AIDS Project, Minneapolis, MN, for their participation in this research. In addition, the authors thank Stephen Asche for his assistance with data analyses and Dan Cambers and Emer Day for their help with data collection.

nities. At the community level, volunteer organizations made up of "everyday people" have taken the lead in educating the public about HIV and offering social support to persons affected by AIDS and persons living with AIDS (PWAs). AIDS service organizations are widespread in the United States, with thousands of volunteers providing emotional, instrumental, and practical support to PWAs through social contacts, advocacy work, resource acquisition, and assistance with tasks of daily living and transportation (Arno, 1986; Chambré, 1991; Kayal, 1993; Omoto & Snyder, 1990, 1993; Ouellette, Cassel, Maslanka, & Wong, 1995; Velentgas, Bynum, & Zierler, 1990; Williams, 1988).

As the number of individuals affected by and infected with HIV continues to increase and as PWAs live longer (Centers for Disease Control and Prevention [CDC], 1996c), volunteers play a critical role in reducing the costs of HIV. Public education provided by volunteers and volunteer programs may help slow the rate of new HIV infections and the costs they entail. In addition, the financial costs of caring for PWAs drop markedly when volunteers provide services that would otherwise be paid for by insurance companies, governmental agencies, and special assistance programs (Hellinger, 1993; Turner, Catania, & Gagnon, 1994). In fact, an increasing reliance on community-based organizations for medical care by PWAs means that AIDS-related deaths have become less likely to take place in inpatient hospital settings and more likely to occur at home or in hospices (Folkman, Chesney, & Christopher-Richards, 1994; Kelly, Chu, & Buehler, 1993). Perhaps more importantly, volunteers can help alleviate some of the psychological toll that HIV disease exacts from PWAs and their social networks. AIDS volunteers may buffer PWAs and people close to them from many of the stressors that a long and unpredictable illness such as HIV disease presents. Volunteers may also help PWAs and their social networks to find new meaning in their lives and to surmount challenges posed by living with HIV, including changed physical capabilities and stigmatization by others.

In light of the significant contributions AIDS volunteers make in confronting the HIV epidemic, it is important to better understand the ways in which the structures and programs of AIDS organizations affect PWAs (see Chapter 7) as well as the dynamics of the relationships between PWAs and their volunteer "buddies." In this chapter, we will describe the context in which volunteer-PWA relationships develop and the factors that make them unique from other relationships. In addition, using data, we will examine volunteer expectations and perceptions for their relationships with client PWAs, and we will consider the connections between closeness in these relationships and volunteer perceptions of satisfaction with their work, relationship quality, and stress.

■ The Context of Volunteer-PWA Relationships

Common among the services provided by AIDS organizations are "buddy" programs in which one or more volunteers are paired to work with eligible client PWAs. Organizations recruit community members for buddy programs, inform them about HIV and train them in communication and assistance skills, assign them to work with specific client PWAs, and monitor their performance. Because PWAs may lack or lose many of their traditional sources of social support (Hays, Chauncey, & Tobey, 1990; Johnston, Stall, & Smith, 1995; Kurdek & Schmitt, 1987; McCann & Wadsworth, 1992; Pearlin, Mullan, Aneshensel, Wardlaw, & Harrington, 1994; Raveis & Siegel, 1991), they turn to AIDS service organizations for assistance in meeting their social, emotional, and practical needs. Volunteer buddies are trained to anticipate, recognize, and respond to these needs. As such, they bring specialized knowledge of HIV disease and available resources to their relationship with a client PWA and they contribute to the development and maintenance of that relationship by assisting with mundane tasks and providing emotional support.

Volunteers generally initiate contact with AIDS organizations after having learned about their programs from people they know who are volunteers or affected by HIV or through newspapers or public service announcements (Snyder & Omoto, 1992). They may seek out AIDS volunteer work for a variety of reasons (Omoto & Crain, 1995a; Omoto & Snyder, 1993, 1995). Some volunteers are motivated by a desire to feel good about themselves, some wish to help their community, some join friends already volunteering, some simply want to learn more about HIV disease, and some may hope to alleviate concerns about their own health and gain a sense of control over their own disease.

Once involved, AIDS service organizations typically ask volunteer buddies to make commitments to provide assistance to one or more

PWAs for a considerable period of time (often 6 months or more) and at sometimes sizable personal cost (Omoto & Snyder, 1995). These costs involve time, money, and resources to be sure, but unlike many other forms of community service, they include perceptions of stigmatization from others (Omoto & Crain, 1995b; Omoto, Snyder, & Crain, 1998; Snyder, Omoto, & Crain, 1996; see also Chapter 2). Volunteers make these tremendous commitments and endure these costs without any legal or normative obligation to their future client, who, at the beginning of their work, is someone whom they have never even met.

Meanwhile, PWAs may have very different reasons for approaching an AIDS organization and asking for help. Some may need one-time assistance locating medical and financial resources or handling insurance problems. Others may seek long-term assistance from a case manager who can coordinate the services of a team of health care professionals. Even among PWAs who contact an AIDS service agency to participate in a buddy program, there may be numerous and overlapping motivations. Some PWAs may feel that members of their existing social network are unable to provide appropriate resources or support. Other members of a PWA's social network may become so overly sensitive to the needs and demands of HIV disease that interactions with them are stressful for PWAs, or the disease comes to redefine their relationship (Crandall & Coleman, 1992). Some PWAs may also simply want to protect their family and friends from feelings of obligation for meeting their increasing needs or from the stress of their illness.

Clearly, the support relationship that develops between volunteer buddies and client PWAs is qualitatively different from those most commonly described in the interpersonal relationships literature. Because of this, most theories of attraction and relationship initiation must be stretched to accommodate volunteer-PWA relationships. Consider, for example, the research literature on friendship. Traditional views of friendship suggest that physical proximity, familiarity, and perceived similarity are essential for initial attraction (Berscheid, 1985; Brehm, 1992; Fehr, 1996). Theoretically, people who are geographically close to one another will grow increasingly familiar with each other and, if they perceive common interests and abilities, will continue to develop mutually positive feelings. Attraction is further strengthened by reciprocity of liking, perceptions of equity, and the sharing of direct rewards (Brehm, 1992).

One way in which volunteer-PWA relationships are likely to differ from such "traditional" relationships is in the expectations with which participants enter them. Volunteers may expect to provide assistance and support to PWAs without concern for reciprocity or equity (see van Yperen, Buunk, & Schaufeli, 1992, for a similar argument regarding individual differences between nurses). There is also likely to be some dissimilarity between volunteers and PWAs in skills and capabilities, with PWAs tending to have less stamina, physical strength, and greater psychological need than volunteers. The usual patterns of reciprocal disclosure (Cunningham, Strassberg, & Haas, 1986) may also be disrupted to start with because volunteers often know more about their client PWA, including the highly sensitive information that they are HIV positive, than the PWA knows about the volunteer. Volunteers may enter these relationships with a highly romanticized notion of what their work will be like, focusing on the good work that they will selflessly do and underestimating the stress they are likely to encounter in caring for someone with HIV disease.

In addition to expectations, the development of volunteer-PWA relationships and what "pushes" the growth of these relationships may differ from other interpersonal relationships. Volunteer-PWA relationships develop in a context that includes the stress of a progressive disease and the possible death of one member of the pair. Most AIDS organizations do not have systematic methods of pairing volunteer buddies with PWAs. Rather, a case manager or client services director makes a "best guess" about who will be a good match for whom so that volunteer-PWA relationships develop between more or less randomly paired individuals. After initial introductions, it is also generally up to the individuals to negotiate their relationship. Consequently, volunteers and PWAs may have little in common beyond their mutual involvement in the AIDS organization prior to meeting, and the impetus for initiating their relationship is likely to focus on managing the client's disease and meeting his or her needs. For these reasons, the course of the client's disease may have a significant impact on how the relationship develops. Responding to the client's needs may require that volunteers and PWAs spend more time together, do more diverse activities together, and strengthen their impact on each other when the client is very ill. When the disease remits, the PWA may be less needy and may even withdraw from the relationship. Thus, HIV disease may influence interdependencies between the volunteers and PWAs by determining the nature of their interactions (see Thibaut & Kelley, 1958).

As the behavioral interdependence in volunteer-PWA relationships changes over its development and the course of the PWA's disease, volunteer perceptions of their satisfaction with their work, the quality of their relationship with the PWA, and the stress from this relationship may be affected. Interdependence between volunteers and PWAs may mutually benefit relationship participants. For example, the volunteer and relationship may fulfill the PWA's needs for companionship, social support, and practical assistance. At the same time, the relationship may provide volunteers with avenues for expressing their values, learning new skills, and enhancing their self-esteem. To the extent that behavioral interdependence promotes fulfillment of these goals, volunteers and PWAs should feel positive affect toward each other and their relationship. In general, then, greater interdependence, or closeness, should be associated with greater satisfaction with the relationship and perceptions of higher quality relationships. This should be true especially for relationships in which closeness increases relative to those that stagnate or dissolve. Thus, increases in closeness over time should be associated with positive changes in perceptions of the volunteer-PWA relationship.

Closeness between two people who face the possible early death of one as well as general social stigmatization is also likely to involve a great deal of stress. More so than other types of relationships, volunteer-PWA relationships are likely to be ones in which emotionally volatile issues such as death, disfigurement, and declining capabilities are explicitly or implicitly addressed. As such, increasing closeness may result in both relationship participants feeling emotionally exhausted or stressed. In addition to a positive relationship between closeness and satisfaction and relationship quality, therefore, a similar association between closeness and stress may be expected in these relationships.

Clearly, there may also be liabilities for volunteers in developing overly close relationships with PWAs. Too much perceived similarity to a client or too much closeness may be psychologically detrimental for a volunteer, given the likelihood of how the relationship will end. When people care about others who are in trouble, they may experience some of the distress of the situation (Hobfoll & London, 1986). Volunteers who feel especially similar or close to PWAs with whom they work, compared to volunteers who perceive less similarity or closeness, may be particularly vulnerable to stress as their client's health changes, and they may experience a decline in their own psychological well-being when the client is ill. It is possible, then, that very close volunteer-PWA relationships will actually be marked by decreased satisfaction, lessened relationship quality, and increased stress.

As we have suggested, volunteer-PWA relationships have several unique features that distinguish them from the interpersonal relationships that are the focus of much of the research literature. Yet, these relationships are important potential sources of strength and stress for both of their participants. To empirically address some of the issues our analysis has raised, therefore, we turned to a longitudinal study of AIDS volunteerism. The data we present are particularly appropriate because they were collected from buddy volunteers over the course of their relationships with client PWAs and therefore capture some of the dynamic characteristics of volunteer-PWA relationships.

We will first examine the nature of volunteer expectations and beliefs about their buddy relationships during training and before they were assigned to client PWAs. We expected that volunteers might idealize these relationships at the outset, leaving them disappointed and dissatisfied once the reality of their work became clear. We will also examine how the closeness of the volunteer-PWA relationship affects volunteer evaluations of these relationships and the satisfaction and stress they perceive from their work. In general, we expected relationship closeness to be related to perceptions of better relationships and more satisfying and less stressful work.

▓ A Study of Volunteer-PWA Relationships

The data on which we draw come from a longitudinal study of AIDS volunteers that is part of a larger program of research on AIDS volunteerism (see Omoto & Snyder, 1995). In conducting this research, individuals who contacted one of three AIDS service organizations in the midwestern region of the United States and expressed interest in becoming a volunteer were informed about the opportunity to participate in the study. Volunteers who agreed to participate completed a questionnaire about their upcoming volunteer experiences prior to an orientation and training session at their organization. After training, volunteers completed another questionnaire before being assigned to a client PWA (that is, as a buddy) by the organization. Volunteers who were assigned to provide direct support services for a PWA were sent a third questionnaire 3 months after their assignment and a fourth questionnaire 3 months later (a total of 6 months into their relationship with the PWA). The latter two questionnaires focused primarily on aspects of the volunteer's relationship with the client PWA. Volunteers received monetary payment for each of the questionnaires they completed and questionnaires were matched over time through the use of random identification codes.

A subsample of 167 volunteers who completed all four of the questionnaires was selected for the analyses reported here. All of these individuals had elected to serve as buddy volunteers and were actually assigned to work with a client. In addition, we focused on only those volunteers who successfully completed 6 months of service with at least one primary client and whose last two questionnaires referenced the same client relationship. Some volunteers were assigned to multiple or sequential clients for several reasons, including poor match with the client, death of a client, or a request for reassignment from either the volunteer or client. By examining only those volunteers who worked with the same client over a 6-month period, we could insure the continuity of their responses, an essential condition for testing many of our hypotheses.

This sample of volunteers included 94 women and 73 men ranging in age from 17 to 61 years; the average age was 35.9 years. Most participants were white (95%) and well educated; 89% reported having attended at least some college and 56% had earned at least a baccalaureate degree. Median household income among these volunteers was about $30,000, and the majority (70%) reported working 40 or more hours per week in paid employment. Although 38% of volunteers were not dating at all, 5% were dating more than one person, 15% maintained an exclusive dating relationship, and 40% maintained a cohabiting relationship with their spouse or partner. Volunteers most commonly described themselves as heterosexual (49%), although many reported being homosexual (43%) or bisexual (8%). About half (51%) were willing to report that they had been tested for HIV antibodies prior to volunteering at their AIDS organization.

In the pretraining questionnaire, we asked volunteers what they thought their volunteer work would be like. Volunteers rated their expectations for their upcoming volunteer work as well as what they thought their relationship with a client would be like. Using 7-point scales (1 = *not at all*, 7 = *extremely*), volunteers rated the extent to which they thought a series of adjectives would describe their volunteer work. Based on preliminary analyses, we created an index of volunteer *satisfaction* by summing over and averaging the ratings of a cluster of nine adjectives (e.g., satisfying, rewarding, exciting).

Participants also rated how close they thought they would be to their client as well as how emotionally invested they would be in their volunteer-PWA relationship, how important the relationship would be to them personally, and how satisfied they expected to be with it. The ratings of closeness, emotional investment, importance, and satisfaction were highly intercorrelated and combined into a composite measure of expected *relationship quality*.

In addition, participants rated how similar they thought they would be to their client on eight attributes (e.g., "educational level," "attitudes, values, and beliefs"). These were combined to create a measure of expected *similarity*.

The measures described above were collected when volunteers first contacted their agencies prior to training or meeting their PWA buddies. Hence, these responses were used to examine volunteer expectations. Later, volunteers completed identical measures of satisfaction, relationship quality, and similarity after having worked as a buddy for 3 months and then again after a total of 6 months of service. These later questionnaires were used to assess the development of volunteer-PWA relationships. Also included in the later questionnaires, but not included among the expectation measures, was a single question about relationship *stress* in which participants rated the stressfulness of their relationship with their client.

Taken together, then, measures of satisfaction, relationship quality, and similarity to a client PWA were completed by volunteers before they became active and after they had worked as a buddy for several months. A measure of stress was also available but only from the 3 and 6 month assessments. Descriptive information for each of these measures at each time period can be found in Table 6.1.

TABLE 6.1 Means and Standard Deviations for Pre- and Postassignment Satisfaction, Relationship Quality, Similarity, Stress, and Closeness

| | Preassignment Expectations | | Postassignment Expectations | | | |
| | | | 3-Month Perceptions | | 6-Month Perceptions | |
	Mean	Standard Deviation	Mean	Standard Deviation	Mean	Standard Deviation
Satisfaction	5.80	.66	5.40	.90	5.24	1.04
Relationship quality	5.42	.75	4.70	1.18	4.71	1.28
Similarity	3.75	.77	3.36	1.04	3.25	1.08
Stress			2.83	1.53	3.28	1.65
Closeness[a]			.00	2.23	.00	2.16

NOTE: Higher numbers indicate greater satisfaction, relationship quality, similarity, stress, and closeness.
a. Closeness was computed as the sum of three standardized indicators, including the number of contacts and amount of time spent with the client, the number of different activities engaged in with the client, and the amount of perceived influence from the client.

Expectations of AIDS Volunteers

We began by examining volunteer expectations for their work and relationship with a PWA and the extent to which these expectations were realized after several months of service. In general, volunteer experiences fell short of expectations at both the 3- and 6-month follow-ups. For example, as Table 6.1 shows, volunteer ratings of satisfaction with their work before training (column 1) were higher than their reports of satisfaction after 3 months (column 3) and after 6 months (column 5). In fact, statistical comparisons of the later reports to the expectation ratings revealed significant differences, $ts > 5.60$, $ps < .001$. In addition, volunteer reports of satisfaction were higher earlier in their experiences than later; the statistical comparison of the 3- versus 6-month ratings was significant, $t(165) = 2.91$, $p < .01$. Thus, volunteers' satisfaction with their work was less than they had expected and also declined over the course of their relationships with PWAs. Similarly, volunteers' expectations about the quality of the relationships they would have with their client PWAs were significantly higher than their reported relationship quality at either 3 months or at 6 months (statistical comparison $ts > 7.20$, $ps < .001$), although these latter two ratings were not significantly different from each other.

Volunteers also expected to be more similar to their client PWA prior to meeting than after knowing this person for either 3 or 6 months, $ts > 4.50$, $ps < .001$. Similarity ratings were also significantly higher earlier in the relationships than later, $t(163) = 2.03$, $p < .05$. In short, volunteers perceived less actual similarity to their client PWAs than they had anticipated, and these perceptions of relative dissimilarity continued to increase as their relationships continued. It is not clear, of course, if this increasing dissimilarity was the result of volunteers getting to know their client PWAs better over time, an accurate reflection of changes over time, or even a way that volunteers may have psychologically distanced themselves from client PWAs. Suffice it to say, volunteers' perceptions of what their actual experiences as buddies were like did not live up to their preassignment expectations across a variety of different dimensions.

Closeness of Volunteer-PWA Relationships

Beyond knowing that volunteers entered into their relationships with client PWAs with relatively high expectations that were not fulfilled, however, we were especially interested in the nature of the relationships that developed. In particular, we were interested in investigating how the closeness of these relationships might be related to volunteers' satisfaction with their work, perceived relationship quality, and relationship stress.

Relationship closeness can be conceptualized as the frequency, diversity, and strength of the impact that relationship partners have on each other (see Berscheid, Snyder, & Omoto, 1989a; Kelley et al., 1983). Together, indices of impact across these three dimensions can be obtained by asking relationship members to report on the activities they do and time they spend with each other. That is, closeness should be revealed in the patterns of interdependence inherent in the activities shared by relationship partners (Berscheid, Snyder, & Omoto, 1989b). Thus, in both the 3- and 6-month questionnaires we asked volunteers to complete several indices of behavior that are conceptually related to patterns of closeness. Specifically, volunteers reported on the number of contacts and amount of time they spent with their client in a typical week, the number of different activities they had engaged in with their client, and the amount of influence they felt their client had on them. These measures were patterned after research on relationship closeness (Berscheid et al., 1989b) and provided information on patterns of behavioral interdependence in volunteer-PWA relationships. To create a three-component indicator of relationship closeness, therefore, we standardized and summed these different measures of contact, time, and influence.

To examine the associations between closeness and the other variables of interest, we conducted analyses in which we attempted to predict volunteer satisfaction, relationship quality, and stress from relationship closeness at both the 3- and 6-month assessment points. Specifically, we used hierarchical multiple regression techniques in which relationship closeness was entered as the first step in a prediction equation. Because of the possibility that extremely close volunteer-PWA relationships might actually prove more burdensome, difficult, and painful, we added a second step to these analyses in which we tested for curvilinear associations between closeness and the other measures. If increasing closeness predicts changes in satisfaction, relationship quality, or stress that are noncontinuous or nonlinear (e.g., slight increases followed by more rapid increases or decreases), then adding a quadratic term should significantly increase the predictive power of our equation (Cohen & Cohen,

1983). Thus, our general analysis strategy was to enter closeness first to assess its linear association with each outcome measure followed by a quadratic term (computed by squaring the closeness measure) to test for nonlinear trends. In all cases, statistical tests of our overall prediction equations were significant, indicating that closeness was meaningfully related to each of the outcomes, $Fs > 8.20$, $ps < .001$. In what follows, therefore, we more carefully examine the pictures of volunteer-PWA relationships that emerge over time as a function of closeness.

Impact of Closeness on Volunteer-PWA Relationships at 3 Months. Relatively early in volunteer-PWA relationships, volunteer satisfaction was simply and linearly related to relationship closeness, with greater closeness predicting greater satisfaction. In addition, however, the test of the curvilinear relationship between these variables was also significant, $Fs > 3.80$, $ps < .05$. Although volunteer satisfaction tended to increase along with relationship closeness, it began to level off at the highest levels of closeness.

A similar pattern of results was found in the analysis of relationship quality. In this case, closeness had both linear and curvilinear relationships with quality, $Fs > 4.90$, $ps < .05$. Volunteer perceptions of relationship quality increased as closeness increased, although there was a tendency for quality to level off at the highest levels of closeness. As with satisfaction, then, increasing closeness was generally associated with increasing relationship quality, although the closest relationships were not rated as of higher quality than moderately close ones. This pattern of results suggests that increasing relationship closeness may not always benefit volunteers in their work with PWAs. Very close relationships were associated with levels of satisfaction and relationship quality that were similar to moderately close relationships.

Interestingly, this curvilinear relationship was again obtained when volunteers' reports of stress in their helping relationships were examined as a function of relationship closeness, $Fs > 3.60$, $ps < .06$. Of particular note here, however, is the fact that the pattern of association between closeness and stress was exactly the same as for satisfaction and relationship quality instead of being inverse. That is, volunteers who reported moderate levels of closeness experienced the most stress in their relationships, and those who reported relatively low closeness perceived the least stress. Increasing closeness was generally related to increasing stress except at high levels, where perceptions of stress actually showed a slight decrease.

The picture that emerges from the 3-month cross-sectional data, therefore, is one in which moderate to high levels of closeness are related to greater satisfaction, higher relationship quality, and increased stress in volunteer-PWA relationships. As closeness reaches relatively high levels —where volunteers report considerable interdependence with their client PWA—these patterns of association begin to level off and even reverse direction. Although the closest relationships were associated with less stress, this was not accompanied by increased satisfaction or relationship quality.

We suggest that the similar pattern of results for satisfaction, relationship quality, and stress may result from what is likely to be a certain amount of ambivalence in volunteer-PWA relationships. These are relationships in which quality and stress may go hand in hand, and both are facilitated by relationship closeness. It is not the case that as relationship closeness and quality increase stress decreases, but rather, stress also increases.

The results may also simply present a snapshot of the process of relationship negotiation in which stress and disagreement are inevitable, and perhaps even necessary, stepping stones to closer, more intimate, and higher quality relationships (Braiker & Kelley, 1979). In addition, they may reflect some of the unique characteristics of volunteer-PWA relationships in which getting closer and having higher quality relationships serves to remind volunteers of the pain, heartache, and stress they may experience when their client is seriously ill, develops new or recurrent symptoms, or dies.

Finally, to rule out the possibility that volunteer expectations were responsible for the obtained results, we examined the potential impact of volunteers' preassignment expectations of satisfaction and relationship quality on our results (there was no preassignment measure of stress). In both cases, preassignment ratings of satisfaction and relationship quality were significantly related to the later 3-month assessments. However, conducting analyses in which expected satisfaction and relationship quality were controlled for before attempting to predict satisfaction and quality from closeness did not alter the pattern of results. For volunteer satisfaction and relationship quality, the reported results were virtually unchanged, and the curvilinear trends continued to obtain, $Fs > 3.30, ps < .07$. Thus, the nature of the associations between closeness and 3-month satisfaction and relationship quality was not due to prior expectations.

Impact of Closeness on Volunteer-PWA Relationships at 6 Months. Volunteer reports of satisfaction, relationship quality, and stress after 6 months of service were analyzed using the same hierarchical multiple regression procedures as described for the 3-month data. In each regression equation, we attempted to predict the outcome measure from the concurrent measure of closeness. Because we had obtained significant curvilinear effects in the early data, we again sequentially tested for both linear and curvilinear associations between closeness and satisfaction, relationship quality, and stress.

As with the 3-month results, closeness was linearly related to volunteer satisfaction at 6 months, $F(1, 164) = 39.66$, $p < .001$, but unlike the earlier results, there was no evidence of additional curvilinear trends. Once volunteers and PWAs had been in relationships together for 6 months, greater closeness was simply and directly related to greater satisfaction with volunteer work. Thus, relatively low levels of closeness were associated with low levels of satisfaction, moderate closeness with moderate satisfaction, and high closeness with relatively high satisfaction. By this time, then, it may be that volunteers and PWAs have more fully negotiated their relationships and have established clear and predictable patterns of interaction or levels of interdependence. The closer these relationships, the more satisfied volunteers are with their work.

Examination of relationship quality after 6 months again showed linear and curvilinear associations with closeness, $Fs > 3.40$, $ps < .06$. Moreover, this pattern of results was the same as for the 3-month measures. Specifically, as closeness increased, volunteers tended to report higher quality relationships. At the highest levels of closeness, however, perceptions of quality began to plateau; volunteers in the closest relationships reported relationships similar in quality to those of volunteers who reported moderately close relationships with their client PWAs.

Unlike the earlier reports of stress, volunteer perceptions of stress in their volunteer-PWA relationships at 6 months were only directly and linearly related to closeness, $F(1, 165) = 15.60$, $p < .001$. Adding a curvilinear component to this equation did not increase its predictive power. Simply put, the highest levels of closeness were related to the highest perceived stress levels. Just as increasing closeness was associated with greater satisfaction, then, it was also related to increasing stress.

Overall, the pattern of associations between volunteer outcomes and closeness in volunteer-PWA relationships at 6 months was simpler than what was obtained in the 3-month assessments. For example, although relationship quality continued to be both linearly and curvilinearly related to closeness (with quality leveling off at high levels of closeness), volunteer satisfaction and stress were more simply and directly related to closeness. Because volunteer expectations prior to training were again related to their corresponding 6-month measures, we repeated the above analyses but after controlling for initial expectations. The 6-month results were virtually identical in these new analyses, meaning that the relationships between closeness and the different volunteer outcomes at 6 months could not be accounted for by the prior expectations of volunteers.

Closeness and the Development of Volunteer-PWA Relationships. Our final set of analyses examined how *changes* in closeness between 3 and 6 months were related to changes in volunteer satisfaction, relationship quality, and perceived stress over this same time period. Our separate analyses of the early and later data indicated that closeness in volunteer-PWA relationships was related to satisfaction, relationship quality, and stress but that the precise nature of these associations depended on the time at which they were assessed. Specifically, the implications of being in a very close relationship relative to a less close one were different at 3 and 6 months. Earlier on, the closest relationships also tended to be marked by dampened levels of satisfaction and relationship quality and less stress. Later, however, high relationship closeness related to high satisfaction, plateauing quality, and relatively high stress.

These different patterns of association may reasonably reflect adjustments made by volunteers to the changing demands of their clients and relationships. Clearly, client PWAs are also likely to change and accommodate their volunteers, but our data do not permit us to directly examine these possibilities. To examine how changes in closeness related to changes in volunteer satisfaction, relationship quality, and stress, we created a residualized measure of change in closeness by using the 3-month closeness scores to predict the 6-month closeness scores. We created similar measures of change in satisfaction, relationship quality, and stress. By way of these residualized change scores, we were able to obtain somewhat stable measures of differences in client-PWA relationships over time. In short, we were able to take full advantage of our longitudinal data and to examine changes over time.

To investigate whether changes in relationship closeness were related to changes in volunteer outcomes, we computed the correlations between pairs of the computed residualized change scores. We found that a positive change in closeness was significantly related to improving volunteer satisfaction, $r = .21, p < .01$. As volunteers and clients became closer, therefore, volunteers derived greater satisfaction from their work. Our earlier analyses indicated that volunteers were not as satisfied with their work as they had expected to be before they began it. Nonetheless, as they actually developed increasingly closer relationships with their client PWAs, they reported greater satisfaction. Clearly, a variety of separate and overlapping explanations can be offered for this correlation, but it is perhaps sufficient to emphasize that it was the *change* in relationship closeness that related to increasing satisfaction among volunteers.

A similar, but even stronger, correlation emerged between change in closeness and change in relationship quality, $r = .42, p < .001$. To the extent that closeness increased over time, it was strongly related to increases in perceived relationship quality. In our previous cross-sectional analyses, these two variables were consistently related to one another but also included significant curvilinear associations. In these longitudinal analyses, however, no evidence for curvilinear trends emerged. There is little published research on changes in closeness, but research on other types of relationships (Berscheid et al., 1989b; Omoto, 1989) suggests that patterns of interdependence are related to judgments of subjectively closer relationships. In these data, we found that even though the quality of volunteer-PWA relationships did not live up to volunteers' expectations for them, as the relationships grew closer over time, volunteers perceived them to be of higher quality.

Finally, the correlation between changes in closeness and changes in stress was small and not significantly different from zero, $r = .06, ns$. It is possible, then, that closeness and perceived stress follow independent developmental tracks in volunteer-PWA relationships. And indeed, we suggested that closeness in these relationships may increase for at least two distinctly different reasons: because PWAs become more seriously ill or because volunteers and PWAs enjoy each other's company. The implications of these two reasons for stress experienced by volunteers are clearly very different. Volunteers who are drawn closer to client PWAs out of health necessity may perceive their relationships to be more stressful than volunteers who develop closer relationships for relatively more intrinsic reasons. Unfortunately, tracking the health status of PWAs was beyond the scope of the present study and remains for future research.

In relating the lack of a correlation between change in closeness and change in stress to our cross-sectional analyses, we had found that closeness and stress were curvilinearly related at 3 but not at 6 months. Early on, high levels of closeness were associated with less stress, whereas later, high levels of closeness were related to greater stress. What may also covary with these changes, of course, is the health of client PWAs. To the extent that volunteers and PWAs are in a relationship together over time, they are likely to encounter increasingly frequent episodes of poor physical and mental health of the PWA (at least under current standards of care). Although closeness may be rewarding and produce perceptions of higher quality relationships and satisfaction, it may also be a liability in such situations. Volunteers who are closer to their client PWA may experience greater stress when that PWA experiences a health decline. This reasoning is supported by the fact that an index of volunteer perceptions of client functioning at 6 months (including ratings of how dependent, emotionally needy, weak, and lonely the client was judged to be) was significantly related to volunteer reports of relationship stress, $r = .26$, $p < .001$. Specifically, the poorer the perceptions of client functioning, the greater the stress reported by the volunteer.

Summary and Conclusions

Volunteers appeared to enter into their buddy relationships with relatively high expectations that ended up being significantly and positively related to several volunteer outcomes after 6 months of service. Unfortunately, the reality of their experiences after entering service did not live up to their expectations. On every measure, the volunteer experience after both 3 and 6 months of service fell below preassignment expectations. Compared to what they anticipated, volunteers found that their work was less satisfying, they had less in common with their client PWA, and their relationships were of lower quality.

Relatively early glimpses of volunteer-PWA relationships, at 3 months, revealed complex associations between closeness and volunteer reports of satisfaction, relationship quality, and stress. These findings suggest that increasing interdependence, in terms of interaction frequency, diversity, and strength of influence, may produce higher quality relationships, at least as perceived by volunteers, but only to a point. For volunteers who reported their relationship with a client to be either relatively low or high in closeness, their perceptions of their work and the quality of their relationships were dampened. Taken at face value, these results suggest that AIDS service organizations may want to consider assigning duties and activities so as to encourage a moderate level of closeness between volunteers and client PWAs, at least relatively early in these relationships.

Volunteers and PWAs are likely to adapt to the demands of the PWA's disease and negotiate a relationship in light of these demands. When illness escalates, the role of the volunteer may expand and include increases in shared time and activities and increased closeness. In fact, changes in closeness were positively correlated with changes in volunteer satisfaction and relationship quality. After 6 months of service with the same PWA, and even after controlling for initial expectations, volunteers who developed relationships relatively low in closeness reported lower quality relationships, little satisfaction with their work, and less stress. For volunteers who developed relatively close relationships, however, perceptions of satisfaction, relationship quality, and relationship stress were also all higher. It is important to note that the present study focused on relationship closeness and the experiences and perceptions of volunteers. A more detailed examination of the impact of PWA health on these relationships and their dynamics remains for future research.

▓ Recommendations for Service Organizations and Directions for Future Research

By all estimates, the number of PWAs will increase in the years ahead as more people become infected with HIV, as those already infected become ill, and as medical advances extend the life expectancy and quality of life of PWAs. Thus, greater numbers of people are likely to seek the services and assistance of AIDS service organizations and AIDS volunteers. As we have suggested, volunteers make commitments to provide instrumental, social, and emotional support to PWAs without first knowing their potential partners and in the absence of many of the keys to attraction that characterize friendships traditionally studied and described in the social science literature. The resulting relationships not only have unique features that distinguish them from other relationships, but as our results indicate, they are also important potential sources of satisfaction and stress for volunteers and, no doubt, PWAs.

The volunteer-PWA relationship has, at least initially, a specific function or focus, namely the PWA's disease. Consequently, the expectations with which volunteers enter these relationships are likely to be quite different from the expectations people have as they enter into other relationships. Also, as the basis for initiating these relationships, the disease may serve to organize many of the activities and experiences of the relationship partners and may set the relationship on a developmental trajectory that differs from many other relationships. Volunteer-PWA relationships develop against a backdrop of stress, stigmatization, and the possibility of premature death, which may further complicate relationship development. This unique relationship context is not yet well understood, but the present research is an initial attempt to explore some of its complex dynamics. We have traced the expectations that volunteers have as they enter volunteer-PWA relationships and the extent to which their experiences actually end up falling short of these expectations. In addition, we have examined the associations between closeness and volunteers' reports of their satisfaction, relationship quality, and stress relatively early and later in their relationships with client PWAs. Changes in closeness over time were related to changes in satisfaction, relationship quality, and stress, and the implications of these patterns of association were discussed. Finally, the effects reported here could not be accounted for by the expectations of volunteers. Thus, the importance of examining volunteer-PWA relationships and the general volunteer process (Omoto & Snyder, 1995; Omoto, Snyder, & Berghuis, 1993) as they unfold over time is underscored by our results.

These findings have additional implications for how AIDS service organizations train and subsequently counsel their buddy volunteers as their relationships with PWAs develop. Even before volunteers are paired with a PWA, for example, it may be fruitful for organization staff members to prepare volunteers by attempting to align their expectations and likely experiences. That is, volunteers should be warned that although being a buddy is a rewarding experience for most people, it is quite possible that it will not live up to the notions and expections that they have and may even prove to be rather stressful at times.

A second note of caution that may prove beneficial for volunteers is that they should not take on too much too quickly in their relationships with client PWAs. Instead of volunteers attempting to force intimacy with their clients early in the relationship, allowing the closeness of the relationship to develop slowly over time may result in more satisfying and higher quality relationships in the long run. Agency personnel may attempt to regulate the degree to which volunteer-PWA relationships become interdependent by arranging structured interactions between volunteers and PWAs early on and then increasingly backing away from structuring these interactions over time.

These recommendations aside, it is important to recognize that the current research tells but one side of the story. Although understanding the perceptions and experiences of AIDS volunteers provides important and useful insights into the dynamics of these relationships, there is a conspicuous silence about PWAs' perspectives on these very same relationships. The PWA's perspective may be quite different from that of the volunteer. For instance, many volunteers may leave the disease, with its stress and stigma, behind them when their duties are done; they may only temporarily experience the stress of AIDS caregiving (e.g., Folkman et al., 1994; Guinan, McCallum, Painter, & Dykes, 1991; Pearlin et al., 1994). The impact on PWAs is likely to be much greater. In fact, interactions with volunteers may even serve to heighten awareness of their disease and its progression. Asking for assistance may also be aversive for PWAs because it makes salient the toll that the disease has taken or is taking and undermines the PWA's sense of self-efficacy and self-esteem (Clark, 1983; Coates, Renzagla, & Embree, 1983). Thus we cannot assume that PWAs would agree with volunteers in their perceptions of these relationships and their dynamics. In particular, PWAs may be very uncomfortable with close volunteer-PWA relationships, revealing inverted patterns of effects to the ones reported here, and this may be even more likely among PWAs maintaining strong social support networks outside their involvement with an AIDS organization.

In addition to examining the volunteer-PWA relationship from the perspective of the volunteer, our focus in this chapter has been on the connections between relationship closeness and volunteers' perceptions of satisfaction, relationship quality, and stress. We have done so because of our interests in patterns of interdependence and because of our desire to examine volunteer-PWA relationships as they are negotiated and develop. Our results speak to the value of this perspective. By using a measure of behavioral interdependence, we were able to examine changes in the subjective consequences of volunteer-PWA relationships.

Of course, however, there are other relationship parameters that could be examined and that may be related to these and other outcomes of interest. The relatively more structural dimension of volunteer-PWA similarity, for example, could be investigated as a determinant of satisfaction, relationship quality, and stress.[1] A good deal of research on interpersonal relationships has also stressed the role of reciprocity in facilitating relationship development and maintenance (Altman, 1973). Relatedly, perceptions of equity (Walster, Walster, & Berscheid, 1978) and the breadth and depth of disclosure (Altman & Taylor, 1973) have been investigated as determinants of relationship growth and decline. We suggested at the outset that volunteer-PWA relationships are unique among interpersonal relationships; the expectations with which participants enter them may differ as most likely do their perceptions of reciprocity, equity, and disclosure. It remains for future research to further investigate the special features of volunteer-PWA relationships as well as their development and implications for volunteer and PWA perceptions of satisfaction, relationship quality, and stress.

Ultimately, volunteer-PWA relationships are also embedded in the social networks of both volunteers and PWAs. We have suggested that PWAs may seek the assistance of volunteers out of concern for or even to avoid their social networks. Similarly, we have alluded to the fact that volunteers may experience numerous costs from doing AIDS work, one of which may be stigmatization and negative affect (e.g., disapproval, hostility) directed at them from members of their own social networks (see Omoto et al., 1998; Snyder, Omoto, & Crain, 1996, 1997). The extent to which volunteer-PWA relationships conflict with or complement the existing relationships of both participants raises a number of intriguing issues that are also likely to have profound implications for how volunteers and PWAs view their relationships and their relative rewards and costs.

In conclusion, we have attempted to describe the characteristics that distinguish volunteer-PWA relationships from those that are more frequently treated in the interpersonal relationships literature and then to track the development of these relationships. The data we have presented, collected from volunteer buddies as their relationships with PWA clients developed over time, have highlighted the expectations and experiences of volunteers. Furthermore, our examination of the associations between relationship closeness and several outcome measures has illustrated the advantages and liabilities of developing close relationships with PWAs as well as the complex development of such relationships. Volunteer-PWA relationships represent but one type of voluntary helping relationship and only one way in which individuals have taken it upon themselves to do something about HIV. As the HIV epidemic continues to alter the lives of individuals, communities, and the nation, however, these relationships deserve greater systematic research attention. Ultimately, an increased understanding of volunteer-PWA relationships is sure to advance theory on interpersonal processes. In addition, such an understanding will provide numerous practical benefits for AIDS service organizations, and for volunteers and PWAs, in providing better services.

▨ Note

1. In fact, we conducted analyses using similarity instead of closeness to predict volunteer satisfaction, relationship quality, and stress. In general, greater similarity was related to more positive outcomes, although these results were not entirely consistent with our closeness analyses. At 3 months, greater similarity was significantly and positively associated with satisfaction and relationship quality, $Fs > 31.0$, $ps < .001$, and marginally related to less stress, $F = 2.91$, $p < .10$. Similar and significant direct relationships emerged in analyses of the 6-month data, $Fs > 9.90$, $ps < .001$. Unlike the closeness analyses, only one significant curvilinear trend was obtained in the two sets of analyses: 6-month satisfaction increased and then leveled off with increasing similarity, $F(1, 161) = 5.25$, $p < .05$.

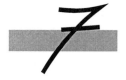

Living Together With AIDS
Social Support Processes in a Residential Facility

LAWRENCE R. FREY
JIM L. QUERY, Jr.
Loyola University Chicago

LYLE J. FLINT
Ball State University

MARA B. ADELMAN
Seattle University

There can be little doubt that people with AIDS (PWAs) are in need of a tremendous amount of social support. As Adelman and Frey (1997) explained:

> Considering the physical devastation, uncertain symptomology, and om-
> nipresent sense of impending death associated with this disease; the loss
> of significant others to AIDS and the fragile social networks left behind
> for those still living with it; and the societal stigma associated with AIDS
> that often results in the loss of social support; no other group of people
> may have more need for community than those affected by AIDS. (p. 5)

PWAs need social support to restore self-esteem, to create meaning during the crisis, and to gain control over their lives.

Given the importance of social support for PWAs, perhaps what is most insidious about this disease is the collapse of traditional institutions and systems that are supposed to provide such support (see Dane & Miller, 1992). Institutions such as the health care system, churches, schools, and businesses have generally failed to adequately address the unique needs of PWAs.

The failure of these social institutions is, in part, a result of the stigma attached to AIDS (see Chapter 2). The AIDS pandemic has been exacerbated by "moralizing" the disease in terms of "innocent or guilty" victims (Teguis, 1992) and by policymakers who view the mention of the disease as taboo. Mainstream perceptions of PWAs are so problematic that "perhaps the single, most important psychological phenomenon associated with the acquired immune deficiency syndrome (AIDS) is the stigmatization that accompanies the disease" (Crandall & Coleman, 1992, p. 163). It thus should come as no surprise that representatives of mainstream institutions often respond negatively to PWAs; even nurses and doctors—who should know much about AIDS—respond irrationally to PWAs (see Klonoff & Ewers, 1990; Norton, Schwartzbaum, & Wheat, 1990).

Given the failure of various macrostructures to meet the needs of PWAs, PWAs must often rely on the "healing web" (Pilisuk & Parks, 1986), "the constellation of informal caregivers—community members, kin, and lovers or friends who provide social support" (Adelman, 1989, p. 31). Unfortunately, loss of support from informal caregivers is all too common. In the case of family systems, for example, although AIDS is sometimes a catalyst for pulling a family together (see Kaisch & Anton-Culver, 1989), loss of social support from family members is far more common (see Metts, Manns, & Kruzic, 1996). The majority of PWAs surveyed felt that their family was not very close or warm (Donlou, Wolcott, Gottlieb, & Landsverk, 1985), had minimal or no contact with their family (Christ, Wiener, & Moynihan, 1986), and had been rejected by at least one family member (Weitz, 1990). Even in families with strong bonds, sons and daughters with AIDS are often abandoned.

The same problems that lead to the lack of family support can be generalized to the availability of support from PWAs' social and personal networks (see Metts et al., 1996; Weitz, 1990). But there is also the fact that, especially in the gay communities, whole social networks have been decimated, thereby wiping out what support there may be: "No other illness in recent memory in the United States has resulted in mourners who grieve not only for the loss of their friends, family, and lovers, but also for their own lives" (Adelman & Frey, 1997, p. 6).

In spite, or more likely because, of the collapse of traditional support systems, PWAs often turn to one another for social support. Gay communities in particular have reframed the ostracization and rejection they have received from mainstream society as an impetus for self-help. As the National Research Council (U.S.) Panel on Monitoring the Social Impact of the AIDS Epidemic (1993) reported, "Already stigmatized by homophobia, distrustful of governmental intrusions and angry over the slowness of those same government agencies to take action, the gay community quickly began to organize volunteer efforts to help their own" (p. 158). By 1983, 2 years after the diagnosis of "Patient Zero," the person responsible for bringing AIDS to the United States (see Shilts, 1987), 45 self-help groups had formed in the United States (Chambré, 1989). By 1991, over 600 community-based AIDS service-providing organizations had been established (National Research Council, 1993).

These alternative types of social support systems have been described as "mediating structures" that bridge (mediate) the gaps between societal institutions (such as government and hospitals) and individuals (such as those with AIDS) (Levin & Idler, 1981). These new models of health care and social support are becoming more widespread, but little is known about whether and how people benefit from them. In a time of tightening budgets for health care, it is crucial that we seek answers to this question.

Our chapter begins to address this issue by examining the effects of formal and informal social support processes within an innovative mediating structure of a residential facility for PWAs. We first examine the nature of mediating structures and how they provide members with social support. We then test predictions concerning the effects of formal and informal social support on perceived health behaviors and satisfaction with living in this residence. The chapter concludes with a discussion of the implications of the findings.

▨ The Nature of Mediating Structures

A mediating structure is an organization or institution that stands between the individual and the macrostructures of society. Mediating structures have two faces: one directed toward their individual members and a "public face that represents an identifiable social group which can be named (and even categorized) by the bureaucracy and which commands a certain amount of economic, political, or moral power" (Levin & Idler, 1981, p. 6). Examples of mediating structures include neighborhood and community associations, religious groups, and alternative health care organizations (e.g., hospices and residential facilities). The difference among them is primarily structural; some are highly organized and formal and others are loosely organized and informal (see Query & James, 1989).

Mediating structures play an especially important role with regard to health care, influencing members' health by (a) preventing illness through the provision of identity as well as material and emotional support; (b) functioning as a channel for information about health care providers, treatment regimens, and health promotion; and (c) offering alternative definitions of illness (Levin & Idler, 1981). Committed to their members' well-being, these organizations and institutions engage in communication that crystallizes coping strategies and reduces uncertainty in a relatively nonthreatening manner (see Query & James, 1989).

The mediating structure examined in this study is a residential facility for people with AIDS that attempts to fill the current gaps in housing, health care, and social support. As a mediating structure, this residence addresses the needs of individual residents and is also responsive and responsible to larger macrostructures (e.g., federal and state governments and funding agencies). In this study, we focus on how the provision of social support in this house affects health behaviors of residents and their satisfaction with group living.

▣ Social Support Processes in Mediating Structures

Mediating structures generally facilitate the provision of social support in two ways: (a) *formal support*, such as weekly support groups; and (b) *informal support*, such as providing opportunities for members to develop a network of interpersonal relationships. Both forms of support are viewed in this study as communicative phenomena in that they are created and sustained through interaction among people (see Albrecht & Adelman, 1987a; Burleson, Albrecht, Goldsmith, & Sarason, 1994).

In the residential facility for PWAs that we study, formal social support is offered via weekly support groups (which every resident must attend for the first 6 weeks of residency; thereafter, they are voluntary), a buddy system (in which newcomers are paired with veteran residents who show them the ropes), in-house educational seminars, social events sponsored by the house, religious/spiritual assistance, and collective bereavement rituals. Informal social support, by contrast, depends on the extent to which residents form strong, close relationships with other residents with whom they can talk about problems, share feelings, and the like when needed. The following discussions examine these formal and informal social support processes and articulate the hypotheses for this study.

Formal Social Support Processes: Support Groups

We focus specifically on support groups because they provide powerful communicative opportunities for individuals to regain a sense of self, community, and control during catastrophic illnesses such as AIDS. Indeed, Hoffman (1991) maintains that support groups are "the single most important and effective intervention for many HIV-infected individuals" (p. 496). In theory, support groups help PWAs "normalize" the effects of this life crisis, recognize fear as a common reaction, provide a place to ventilate emotional reactions, and gain a feeling of control (see Cawyer & Smith-Dupré, 1995; Kelly & Sykes, 1989; Taylor, Falke, Mazel, & Hilsberg, 1988). Maione and McKee (1987) report that professional AIDS counselors believe that "support groups seem to be the most viable way to assist these people [PWAs] in coping with their daily functioning" (p. 20). Unfortunately, few investigations have assessed the effects of support groups on coping with AIDS. Indeed, there are only two recent studies of HIV/AIDS support groups of which we are aware.

Cawyer and Smith-Dupré (1995) conducted an ethnographic study to describe the supportive episodes that occurred during the meetings of an HIV/AIDS support group for health care providers; family members, friends, and lovers of PWAs; individuals who had lost a loved one to the disease; and individuals who were seropositive or infected with AIDS. This group met on a weekly basis, usually for 2 hours, with 3 to 10 members attending each meeting. The authors found that this support group did help people express frustration and other emotions, prepare for complications of the disease and death, and mobilize their energies toward social change. Cawyer and Smith-Dupré concluded that "communicative episodes perform functions integral to the group's success in dealing with issues surrounding AIDS and HIV" (p. 254).

Daniolos (1994) also examined the messages exchanged in a support group of PWAs who lived in a residential facility—the AIDS Community Residence Association House. This support group was initiated in late 1991 and met periodically for about 1 hour during the following 18 months. The group was a microcosm of the house; at various times, it comprised males and females; homosexuals, heterosexuals, and bisexuals; and intravenous drug users. The common themes identified in the messages exchanged in this support group included invasion, rejection, loss, and ambivalence.

The studies by Cawyer and Smith-Dupré (1995) and Daniolos (1994) provide insight into the communicative processes that characterize support groups for PWAs, but they do not examine empirically how participation in and perceived efficacy of support groups shape a variety of outcomes for PWAs (e.g., health practices and satisfaction). Available literature from several relevant contexts, such as Alcoholics Anonymous (Hurt, 1989) and people with cancer (see review by Taylor & Dakof, 1987), however, reveals the beneficial effects of social support.

Lest we fall into the trap of being pollyannaish about social support, let it be said that there can be a debilitating or "dark" side of social support (see Albrecht & Adelman, 1987b; Goldsmith, 1992; La Gaipa, 1990). Social support may come at a price, such as becoming indebted to a person, or may result in negative effects, such as increased stigmatization or loss of control or autonomy (see Goldsmith, 1994). This problematic side of social support is especially important in residential settings for PWAs. Well-intentioned messages do not always have the intended effect. Simple gestures of inquiring about another's health may be viewed as unwanted solicitousness. Physical expressions of affection require sensitivity to personal preferences and knowledge of a person's health status. And a fine line must be walked between helping and pampering so as not to reinforce people's "sick role" (see Adelman & Frey, 1997).

It is by no means clear whether formal social support positively affects residents in such a setting. Indeed, one of the group members in Daniolos's (1994) study, described earlier, fled the residence. One purpose of the present study, therefore, is to assess the effects of the perceived value of formal support processes, in the form of support groups, within an AIDS residence with regard to a variety of perceived health behaviors as well as residents' satisfaction with living in this mediating structure. Based on the literature, the following hypotheses are advanced:

> H1: Residents who experience distinct levels of formal social support within the house demonstrate differences in perceived health behaviors.
>
> H2: Residents who experience distinct levels of formal social support within the house demonstrate differences in the perceived value of group living.

Informal Social Support Processes: Interpersonal Relationships

Informal social support refers to the potential support a person perceives is available from his or her interpersonal relationships. Informal social support is obtained through proactive behaviors on the part of individuals; although mediating structures may facilitate interpersonal relationships, the individual is responsible for developing these connections.

It is generally assumed that social relationships have positive effects on health, but meta-analyses of this relationship have actually found inconsistent effects (e.g., Schwarzer & Leppin, 1989, 1991). The positive benefits seem to be most apparent for seropositive individuals, as a number of studies have found that those who perceive support from family and friends as readily available report less physical distress, hopelessness, and depression (see Metts et al., 1996; Ostrow et al., 1989; Zich & Temoshok, 1987). Schwarzer, Dunkel-Schetter, and Kemeny (1994), for example, conducted a longitudinal study of social support types (informational, tangible, and emotional) and sources (friends, relatives, partners, and organizations) among 587 gay men (45% of whom were seropositive). Participants evaluated the frequency and quality of social support received from these sources for one of eight major stressors ranging from lifestyle changes to general anxiety about AIDS to development of AIDS/ARC in a friend to death from AIDS. The results revealed that friends were the preferred source of social support and that emotional support (e.g., reassuring, listening, and providing advice) was more helpful than informational or tangible support (e.g., taking them to the store). Received social support was also associated with more successful coping across these life stressors.

These findings are consistent with research by O'Brien, Wortman, Kessler, and Joseph (1993), who conducted a year-long study of 637 gay and bisexual men to identify how features of informal relationships, such as social support level and amount and type of conflict, affect particular health attitudes. The results revealed that "perceived availability of support led to reduced symptoms of depression and anxiety" (p. 1165).

The relationship between informal social support and health behaviors has also been shown for those participating in support groups and for those with close ties to the AIDS community. For example, in a study of 52 asymptomatic HIV-positive men and a comparison group of 53 HIV-negative men, Leserman, Perkins, and Evans (1992) hypothesized that "positive coping" was associated with received positive affect and self-esteem and that high social support, operationalized with respect to both participation and satisfaction, would be related to greater levels of coping behaviors. They administered a battery of tests that measured depression, mood, self-esteem, coping behaviors (e.g., maintaining a fighting spirit, planning, personal growth, and seeking social support), satisfaction with support, and participation in AIDS groups. The findings indicated that participation and satisfaction with social support accounted for 69 percent of the variance in the adoption of several positive coping behaviors, including fighting spirit, personal growth, active planning, seeking emotional support, and, to a lesser extent, religious pursuits. Leserman et al. (1992) concluded, "To a large extent, we found that being satisfied with one's social support networks and participating in the AIDS community were related to more healthy coping strategies" (p. 1519). Other studies have reported similar results (see Namir, Alumbaugh, Fawzy, & Wolcott, 1989; Namir, Wolcott, Fawzy, & Alumbaugh, 1987).

Informal social support processes appear to affect the health behaviors of PWAs, but there is a need to test this relationship, as well as the effects of informal support on other outcomes, especially within the context of a mediating structure such as an AIDS residence. The second purpose of the present study, therefore, is to assess the effects of the value of informal support processes within an AIDS residence with regard to residents' perceived health behaviors as well as their satisfaction with living in this mediating structure. Based on the literature, the following hypotheses are advanced:

H3: Residents who experience distinct levels of informal social support within the house demonstrate differences in perceived health behaviors.

H4: Residents who experience distinct levels of informal social support within the house demonstrate differences in the perceived value of group living.

▨ Method

AIDS Residence

The AIDS residence examined here is called Bonaventure House (BH) and is located in Chicago, IL. Established in 1989 by the religious order of the Alexian Brothers of America, BH is one of the largest AIDS residences in the United States, housing 30 residents. There are 13 full-time and 14 part-time staff who provide 24-hour supervision, medical and nursing care, case management (see Budz, 1993), an array of social services, pastoral care (see DiDomenico, 1993), house maintenance, and food preparation. Social support to residents and help with house maintenance and some administrative duties is offered by 150 volunteers.

The mission statement establishes BH as a residential facility for people with AIDS, offering the opportunity for assisted living within a comprehensive supportive environment. Priority is given to applicants who (a) have exhausted all personal resources (family, friends, independent living) and (b) are unable to locate quality housing due to financial limitations imposed by their AIDS-defining illness.

As of November, 1995, BH had housed 274 residents. The average age is between 30-39, but there are residents as young as 20 and as old as 69. Fifty to sixty percent of residents have a history of alcohol or drug abuse, and approximately 25% contracted HIV through intravenous drug use. The average length of stay is 233 days, just over 7 months. Regrettably, 195 (over 71%) of the residents have died since the house opened.

Resident Sample

The current study involves a total of 59 BH residents who answered questionnaires over four time periods: March, 1993; August, 1993; September, 1994; and April, 1995. Each of the 59 residents completed the questionnaire at least once. If residents completed more than one questionnaire, the first one was used.

This sample of residents' ages ranged from 27 to 61, with a mean age of 38.8 (SD = 8.2). The overwhelming majority were male (n = 52), with only 7 being female. Most had resided at BH for 3 months to a year (n = 42), 16 had resided there for less than 3 months, and only 1 had lived there for more than a year. These demographics reflect quite well the total resident population over the past 6 years.

Instrumentation

Adelman and Frey became involved with this house as both volunteers and researchers soon after it opened. Their long-term involvement provided many opportunities to observe the processes and practices that characterize life in this setting. They also conducted in-depth interviews with residents, which subsequently formed the basis for the development of an extensive questionnaire (see Adelman & Frey, 1997).[1] The present study uses portions of the questionnaire that are germane to the effects of formal and informal social support processes on residents' health behaviors and their perceptions of the value of living in this mediating structure. The specific operationalizations of the variables are described below.

Hypothesis 1 predicted a difference in residents' perceived health behaviors on the basis of distinct experiences with formal social support processes in the house. Formal social support was operationalized as residents' perceptions of the value of support group meetings on the following 6-item scale: (a) "Helpful in resolving conflicts among residents"; (b) "Provide me with emotional support"; (c) "Help me deal with the loss of residents"; (d) "Often 'bitch sessions' " (reverse coded); (e) "Ineffective" (reverse coded); and (f) "Enable me to cope better with my illness." Residents responded to each item using a 5-point scale (5 = YES!; 4 = Yes; 3 = ?; 2 = No; 1 = NO!). An analysis of the data demonstrated an internal consistency estimate (Cronbach's alpha) of .83 for this scale. Thirty-third and 67th percentiles were used to divide the sample into three groups corresponding to low (M = 2.16 [all scores are reported on 5-point scale], SD =.48, n = 17), moderate (M = 3.30, SD =.19, n = 18), and high (M = 3.96, SD = .32, n = 20) perceptions of the value of support group meetings. These demarcations enhanced the precision and power of the subsequent statistical tests.

Perceived health behaviors were operationalized as the difference between residents' perceptions of their behavior prior to moving to BH and currently with regard to six behaviors: exercising, dieting, safe-sex practices, spiritual practices, coping well with illness, and socializing with others. Each behavior was responded to along the same 5-point scale described above, first by addressing the question "Did you do the following on a regular basis *before* coming to the BH?" and then the question "Do you *now* do these on a regular basis?" Scores were computed by subtracting former behaviors from current behaviors such that a positive score indicates a perception of engaging more in a behavior after living at BH.

Hypothesis 2 predicted a difference in perceived value of living in this house on the basis of residents' distinct experiences with formal social support processes. The dependent variables relevant to this hypothesis were assessed in two ways. First, to assess residents' general characterization of BH, they responded, using the same 5-point scale, to eight metaphors that they often mentioned in the in-depth interviews conducted with them: home, institution, family, shelter, community, hospital, hotel, and prison. These responses were collapsed into three categories (somewhat similar to Parsons', 1951, taxonomy of organizations): (a) "home," a positively valanced perception, representing the sum of responses to the three items describing BH as a home, family, and community (Cronbach's alpha =.85); (b) "facility," a neutral- to slightly negative-valanced perception, representing the sum of responses to the two items of hospital and hotel (r =.55, p < .001); and (c) "institution," a negatively valanced perception, representing the sum of the responses to the three items of institution, shelter, and prison (Cronbach's alpha =.66). Second, to assess their satisfaction with living at BH, residents responded, using the same 5-point scale, to the following four items: (a) "I am very satisfied living here"; (b) "I am committed to living here"; (c) "I strongly recommend BH to other persons with AIDS"; and (d) "Overall, BH is a positive place to live" (Cronbach's alpha =.88).

Hypothesis 3 predicted a difference in perceived health behaviors on the basis of distinct experiences with informal social support processes in the house; hypothesis 4 predicted a difference in perceived value of living at BH. Informal support was operationalized as residents' perceptions of the availability of social support from their interpersonal relationships in the house, using the same 5-point scale, on the following seven items: (a) "There are people here I can depend on to help me if I really need it"; (b) "There is no one I can turn to here for guidance in times of stress"; (c) "If something went wrong here, no one would come to my assistance" (reverse coded); (d) "I have close relationships here that provide me with a sense of emotional security and well-being"; (e) "There is someone here I could talk to about important decisions in my life"; (f) "There is no one here I can depend on for aid if I really need it" (reverse coded); and (g) "There is no one here with whom I feel comfortable talking to about problems" (reverse coded). This scale resulted in a Cronbach's alpha reliability estimate of .86. Thirty-third and 67th percentiles were used to divide the sample into three groups corresponding to low ($M = 3.21$, $SD = .41$, $n = 19$), moderate ($M = 4.02$, $SD = .13$, $n = 18$), and high ($M = 4.83$, $SD = .23$, $n = 18$) perceptions of informal social support. Hypotheses 3 and 4 used the same dependent variables as the first two hypotheses.

Analysis of the Data

The four hypotheses were tested using four separate three-group MANOVA designs, with formal social support as the independent variable for the first two hypotheses and informal social support as the independent variable for the remaining two hypotheses. The probability level for both multivariate and univariate significance was set at .05.

▨ Results

Formal Social Support Processes

The first hypothesis predicted a difference in perceived health behaviors on the basis of distinct differences in the experience of formal social support (that is, within support groups). Due to incomplete data, several residents were excluded, resulting in a total of 48 individuals for this analysis. The results of the MANOVA provide partial support for the rejection of the null hypothesis, Wilk's Lambda = .60, $F(12, 80) = 1.92$, $p = .040$; observed power = .87, $p = .05$. Two of the 6 health behaviors were significant: exercising, $F(2, 45) = 3.51$, $p = .038$, and safe-sex practices, $F(2, 45) = 3.72$, $p = .032$. A post-hoc Tukey's HSD analysis revealed that the high formal social support group exercised more after living in the house (M = .71, SD = 1.11), whereas the moderate (M = –.28, SD = 1.07) and low formal social support groups (M = –.23, SD = 1.48) exercised less than they had before living in the house. The post-hoc Tukey's HSD procedure showed that the moderate formal social support group practiced safe sex significantly more after living in the house (M = 1.00, SD = 1.28) than the low formal social support group, which actually practiced less safe sex after living in the house (M = –.23, SD = 1.64); the high formal social support group practiced safe sex more after living in the house (M = .12, SD = 1.39) but was not significantly different from the moderate and low formal social support groups.

The second hypothesis predicted a difference in perceived value of the house on the basis of distinct differences in the experience of formal social support. The results of the MANOVA supported the rejection of the null hypothesis, Wilk's Lambda = .58, $F(8, 90)$ = 3.57, p < .001; observed power = .98, p = .05.[2] Three of the 4 variables were found to be significant: home, $F(2, 48)$ = 9.39, p < .001; institution, $F(2, 48)$ = 5.91, p = .005; and satisfaction with BH, $F(2, 48)$ = 12.57, p < .001. The post-hoc Tukey's HSD procedure revealed that the high formal social support group perceived BH to be the positively valanced referent of home (M = 4.22, SD = .63) more than the moderate (M = 3.67, SD = .45) and low (M = 3.08, SD = 1.07) formal social support groups. The high formal support group also perceived BH to be less of the negatively valanced referent of institution (M = 1.84, SD = .74) than the moderate (M = 2.35, SD = .77) and low (M = 2.29, SD = .79) formal social support groups. For satisfaction with BH, the high formal social support group was more satisfied (M = 4.44, SD = .54) than the moderate group (M = 3.93, SD = .51), which was more satisfied than the low group (M = 3.34, SD = .78).

Informal Social Support Processes

The third hypothesis predicted a difference in perceived health behaviors on the basis of distinct differences in the experience of informal social support (that is, via interpersonal contacts). The results of the MANOVA used to test the hypothesis failed to support a rejection of the null hypothesis, Wilk's Lambda = .68, $F(12, 80)$ = 1.41, p = .18; observed power = .72, p = .05.

Hypothesis 4 predicted a difference in the perceived value of the residence on the basis of distinct differences in the experience of informal social support. The results of the MANOVA supported the rejection of the null hypothesis, Wilk's Lambda = .57, $F(8, 90)$ = 3.68, p < .001; observed power = .98, p = .05. Three outcomes were found to be significant: home, $F(2,48)$ = 7.40, p = .002; institution, $F(2, 48)$ = 9.25, p < .001; and satisfaction with BH, $F(2, 48)$ = 6.30, p = .004. The post-hoc analysis revealed that the high informal social support group perceived BH as more of a home (M = 4.29, SD = .47) than both the moderate (M = 3.35, SD = .92) and low (M = 3.39, SD = .47) informal social support groups. The high informal social support group also perceived BH as less of an institution (M = 1.71, SD = .71) than the low (M = 2.39, SD = .71) and moderate (M = 2.71, SD = .64) groups. Finally, the high informal social support group was significantly more satisfied with BH (M = 4.41, SD = .51) than the low group (M = 3.57, SD = .83).

▧ Discussion

For people with HIV/AIDS, adequate health care and social support are often not being met by traditional institutions and/or by networks of family and friends. Fortunately, one of the hallmarks of the AIDS crisis has been the emergence of innovative mediating structures sponsored by grassroot community organizations—from AIDS-awareness educational seminars and support groups to in-home deliveries (e.g., "Meals on Wheels" programs) to residential facilities—that augment informal, personalized support systems and, in some cases, become the sole support and health care delivery to PWAs. However, given the optimization process that is occurring relative to cuts in health care spending, community groups that provide these services are facing the trickle-down effect of restricted state and federal funding and must make difficult decisions about which services will survive. Increasingly, justification for spending is being based on empirical evidence that these mediating structures make a significant difference for those they serve.

The results from this study show that this particular mediating structure—a residential facility—is making a perceived difference in the lives of persons with AIDS. First, Bonaventure House appears to provide residents with high-quality social support. Although residents were divided into high, moderate, and low formal and informal perceived social support groups for the purposes of comparison, the entire sample is very high on a 5-point scale with regard to perceived informal support from interpersonal relationships ($M = 4.01$, $SD = .73$, $n = 55$) and moderate with regard to perceived formal support obtained from support group meetings ($M = 3.18$, $SD = .82$, $n = 55$). This higher rating of the social support from interpersonal relationships versus support groups is significant, $t(53) = 7.17$, $p < .001$, but not surprising, considering that support groups meet only once a week and interpersonal relationships form the basis of daily life in a residential setting. Moreover, of the six conditions (high, moderate, and low with regard to formal and informal social support), only the low formal social support group is on the negative side of the middle point of the scale ($M = 2.16$, $SD = .48$), which suggests that some residents do not perceive themselves as benefiting from support groups. These individuals told us they saw the meetings as "bitch sessions." The remaining groups, however, range from moderate ($M = 3.21$) to very high ($M = 4.83$). Thus, on the whole, Bonaventure House is meeting the goal of offering social support.

Second, the results regarding the effects of social support processes on health behaviors may appear disappointing at first glance, in that differences in informal social support did not affect any of the six outcomes, and differences in formal support only affected exercising and safe-sex practices. Furthermore, although the difference in exercising was in the expected direction, with the high informal social support group exercising more after living in the house than the moderate and low informal social support groups, safe-sex practices showed a difference only between the moderate and the low informal social support groups.[3]

Concluding that social support processes do not affect health behaviors, however, would obscure perhaps the most important health findings from this study: Residents reported that they engaged in significantly more of four of the six health behaviors after living at BH than they did prior to moving there (see Table 7.1). That is, residents said they practiced safe sex more, became more spiritual, coped better with their illness, and socialized more after living at the house than they had prior to living there. The means for the nonsignificant variables of exercise and dieting also increased in this direction. Moreover, when before versus current scores are compared for the high, moderate, and low formal and informal support groups, in all but 6 (out of 36) cases, residents' current health practices for all six behaviors were higher than their

TABLE 7.1   Comparisons of Health Behaviors Before Coming to
Bonaventure House (BH) and Current Behaviors

Variable	n	Behavior Before Coming to BH		Current Behavior		t Value
		Mean	SD	Mean	SD	
Exercising	55	2.91	1.24	2.89	1.29	.10
Dieting	55	2.19	1.00	2.39	1.09	1.33
Safe-sex practices	50	3.59	1.30	3.94	1.21	1.86*
Spiritual practices	55	3.00	1.19	3.43	1.17	3.13**
Coping well with illness	54	3.29	1.13	4.06	.83	5.13***
Socializing with others	53	3.63	1.03	4.07	.80	2.74**

*$p < .05$; **$p < .01$; ***$p < .001$.

health practices prior to living at BH. Bonaventure House thus appears
to have an important effect on residents' perceived health practices.

Third, these same results are mirrored in the findings regarding residents' satisfaction with living at BH. Expected differences were found
with regard to satisfaction with BH and perceptions of BH as a home
and institution on the basis of distinct experiences with both formal and
informal social support. That is, residents with the highest ratings of the
formal social support processes were more satisfied than those who were
in the moderate or low groups, perceiving BH as more of a home (a
positive characteristic) and less of an institution (a negative characteristic). The same finding was also apparent for those with the highest
ratings of the informal social support processes. Clearly, if a resident
takes advantage of the social support processes offered in the house, he
or she is more satisfied with this form of group living. But what seems
most important is that the entire sample, as well as the subsamples com-
prising the six conditions, were very satisfied living at BH, perceiving it
as a home and not an institution. This house thus offers residents the
kind of comfort found in a family home.

These findings are quite remarkable given the problems with collective living at Bonaventure House. Although AIDS is often romanticized
as the "great equalizer" that mysteriously brings people into communion
(see Adelman & Schultz, 1991), the reality is that the diversity, close
proximity, social norms, and house rules pose profound challenges to
offering social support and developing community. Furthermore, in the

midst of coping with their own illness and impending death, residents also face the constant loss of fellow residents (as noted in the Methods section). Offering one another social support in coping with illness and bereavement is tremendously difficult. We find that residents are often caught in a "depression bind": they see themselves in the death of others and must keep some distance so as to "grieve efficiently" when someone passes away if they are to guard against the depression that could compromise their already lowered immune system (see Adelman & Frey, 1994, 1997; Frey, Adelman, & Query, 1996).

The tensions and dilemmas in supporting each other in this unique context cannot be underestimated. Hence, the shifts by residents in their reported health behaviors and the perception of a supportive community at Bonaventure House within the short period of time that they live there are impressive. Perhaps one of the reasons so much is accomplished in this house during this "brief window" is the range of formal and informal social support processes that are available to residents.

This study provides strong and clear empirical evidence of the perceived therapeutic potential of mediating structures like BH.[4] However, whether these findings apply to other residences and other types of mediating structures for people with AIDS or for all the people who rely on such structures (e.g., the elderly) remains to be seen. Of particular concern is that the results of this study are based on self-report methods. Residents are clearly the best judges of how valuable they find the social support processes and their satisfaction with living in the house, but perceived health behavior may not necessarily represent actual behavior. Future studies will need to triangulate perceived health behavior with measures of actual behavior (e.g., number of hours exercised). Future studies would also benefit from having a comparison group to better evaluate the impact of residing versus not residing within such a facility.

There is clearly a great need for health care and social support mediating structures, not just for people with AIDS but for all types of people. These mediating structures are no longer a luxury; they are a necessity. But they are only valuable if they help meet the needs of their members. In the case of Bonaventure House, this residence is perceived by residents as making a significant and important difference in their lives. The value of Bonaventure House is captured poignantly by Maria, one of the residents. Recalling how she felt upon being told that she tested positive for HIV, Maria said,

And I wanted to die at that point. I told them to take all the equipment away from me, and just let me go home and die, but I didn't have a home to go home and die to.

After living at Bonaventure House for awhile, her reflection on what the house means to her speaks volumes: "Understanding and a second family or the family that you never had is here."

▓ Notes

1. The present study is part of an ongoing, longitudinal, social action research program that focuses on how communicative practices help create and sustain community (see Adelman, 1992; Adelman & Frey, 1994, 1997; Adelman, Frey, & Budz, 1994; Adelman & Schultz, 1991; Frey, 1994; Frey & Adelman, 1993; Frey, Adelman, & Query, 1996). The present research team has been together for about 2 years.

2. The results of a Box M test for homogeneity of variance indicated that this assumption had been violated, $\chi^2 = 31.6$, $p = .048$. This violation, however, is of greater concern when group sizes are sharply unequal. Moreover, it can be accounted for in any event by employing a more stringent alpha level (Stevens, 1992). Therefore, even though group sizes are equivalent, Hypothesis 2 was tested at the .01 level of significance. The MANOVA resulting from the test of Hypothesis 2 still provided support for the rejection of the null hypothesis.

3. Given the small sample size of this study, it is tempting to suggest that the lack of significant findings is a result of insufficient power. But in the case of the influence of informal social support on health outcomes, the observed multivariate power was a modest .72.

4. The observed power of the multivariate tests for the three significant hypotheses—.87, .98, and .98, respectively—justifies this conclusion.

Personal Accounts of Disclosing and Concealing HIV-Positive Test Results
Weighing the Benefits and Risks

VALERIAN J. DERLEGA
Old Dominion University

DAVID LOVEJOY
Virginia Consortium Program in Clinical Psychology

BARBARA A. WINSTEAD
Old Dominion University

There is considerable evidence that individuals cope better with stressful events (such as having the human immunodeficiency virus [HIV]) if they have someone with whom to discuss their personal difficulties (Lane & Wegner, 1995; Larson & Chastain, 1990; Ostrow et al., 1989; Pennebaker, 1990). For instance, Remien, Rabkin, Williams, and Katoff (1992)

AUTHORS' NOTE: We are grateful to the clients and staff of various community service organizations in southeastern Virginia for participating in the study. We also thank Jenny Caja at Old Dominion University and undergraduate psychology students at the University of Louisville for preparing transcripts from the original audiotaped interviews. Amy Grimshaw and Susan Sherburne assisted in the development of the coding categories reported in the results. Stephen T. Margulis and Anita Barbee made helpful comments on an earlier draft of the chapter. Lisa Foster from the Virginia Consortium Program in Clinical Psychology participated in conducting the original interviews.

found that having a confidant ("someone around to confide in or talk to about yourself and your problems if you want to," p. 339) was positively associated with psychological coping among persons who were long-term AIDS survivors.

There may be psychological benefits from disclosing HIV seropositivity to others. You may feel accepted, loved, and valued by others even though you are having difficulties; friends and health professionals may be able to provide information and advice in coping with the disease; sexual partners may be able to make more informed decisions about sexual practices and their own risk of contracting the virus (Kalichman, 1995; Wills, 1990). However, revealing information about the diagnosis may also be risky. There is the possibility that disclosure of the HIV diagnosis may lead to rejection and discrimination by others and to emotional distress for loved ones (see Hays et al., 1993; Hoff et al., 1992). Given the potential vulnerability in disclosing HIV seropositivity to others, many individuals who are HIV positive must balance two competing needs: the need to share information about the diagnosis and the need to maintain privacy or control over who, what, and when to tell about the diagnosis (Derlega, Metts, Petronio, & Margulis, 1993; Petronio, 1991).

In privacy regulation, individuals seek to maintain control over the amount and kind of information exchange they have with others. If individuals can exercise control over what they disclose (and how much they say about themselves) to others, then they are maintaining privacy. If others have control over what (and how much) information is known about someone, then individuals have a lower degree of privacy. A key consideration in privacy regulation for HIV-positive individuals is the control of who has access to information about the seropositive diagnosis. Because of the risks associated with self-disclosure (e.g., being rejected, information about the HIV diagnosis being disseminated to unwanted third persons), individuals can exercise control over privacy in part by weighing carefully who to tell about the diagnosis.

In this chapter, we will focus on the reasons why individuals do or do not disclose information about being HIV seropositive after they have learned about their diagnosis. We will also consider how type of target person (e.g., a lover or spouse, parents or siblings, friends, and coworkers) affects the reasons given for disclosure versus nondisclosure. Our assumption is that HIV-positive individuals (like anyone who wishes to maintain privacy) seek to control who has access to the information about the diagnosis. Hence, HIV-seropositive individuals will weigh carefully their reasons for disclosing versus not disclosing information about the diagnosis, which will in turn influence who they actually tell.

Several studies (see Stempel, Moulton, & Moss, 1995, for a recent overview) indicate that HIV-positive individuals select who to inform about the diagnosis. Hays et al. (1993), for instance, examined the self-disclosure of seropositivity to significant others among gay men living in San Francisco. Regardless of the stage of HIV illness (asymptomatic HIV positive [HIV+], symptomatic HIV+, or AIDS diagnosis), men were more likely to disclose their HIV seropositivity to a lover or partner (98%) or a gay friend (95%) than to a family member (sister, 53%; mother, 48%; brother, 43%; father 40%). The men who were asymptomatic were also less likely to disclose the diagnosis to relatives compared to those who had HIV symptoms or who were diagnosed with AIDS.

Perry, Ryan, Fogel, Fishman, and Jacobsberg (1990) also examined disclosure of HIV seropositivity among 40 gay men. The study was limited to whether the men had informed various target persons during the first 3 months after they had been notified of their HIV-seropositive status. Although 52.5% of the men had disclosed to "all present sexual partners" and 67.5% had disclosed to "any friend," only 35% had disclosed to "any family member."

There are a number of reasons why HIV-positive individuals may choose not to disclose their HIV status to others. For instance, Marks, Bundek, et al., 1992, found that gay and bisexual Hispanic men were less likely to inform others about their HIV infection if they had not told these others about their sexual orientation (also see Mason, Marks, Simoni, Ruiz, & Richardson, 1995). Thus, individuals who have not "come out" to others about their sexual orientation may fear the consequences of acknowledging being gay or bisexual if they disclose their HIV seropositivity. Hays et al. (1993) found that, among a sample of gay men, individuals might not disclose their HIV-positive status (especially early in the HIV disease process) to keep family members from worrying about them, to avoid discriminatory treatment at work, to prevent the disruption of personal relationships (e.g., "fear of being misunderstood and having family members draw back," p. 5), or because there would be little or no benefit in disclosing. Mason et al. (1995) also found among Latino and white men that a concern for protecting their parents emotionally was a major consideration in the decision not to disclose to them, even more than a concern for protecting oneself from parents' possible negative reactions.

Disclosure to various sexual partners about having the HIV infection may also reflect judgments about the importance of the relationship, awareness of who can be trusted, and ease of notification, besides reflecting concerns about health risks to past or present sexual partners. Some studies report a high rate of disclosure to an intimate lover, but there is a much lower rate of disclosure to more casual or to past sexual partners (see Hays et al., 1993; Marks, Bundek, et al., 1992; Perry et al., 1994; Perry et al., 1990; Schnell et al., 1992; Stempel et al., 1995). For instance, Perry et al. (1990) found that among gay men who had been notified of their seropositivity in the last three months, 52.5% had informed "all present sexual partners" of their HIV seropositivity; only 10% had informed "any past sexual partner." In particular, gay, bisexual, or heterosexual men who report having multiple sexual partners may be less likely to notify past sexual partners because of the absence of an emotional investment in these relationships or the difficulty in identifying who these partners were if the sexual relations occurred in a casual or anonymous context (Marks, Richardson, Ruiz, & Maldonado, 1992).

Concern about being rejected for an intimate relationship or for sexual relations may play a part in individuals' decisions to avoid or delay disclosing information about their seropositive status to prospective lovers. This fear of being rejected for a relationship is realistic, given that many individuals who are seronegative or who have not been tested for HIV antibodies might prefer to have an intimate relationship with a seronegative partner rather than a seropositive partner (Hoff et al., 1992).

Rationale for Present Research

Issues of self-disclosure are a major concern for individuals diagnosed with the HIV infection, but only a few studies have systematically examined the reasons given by HIV-positive individuals for disclosing versus not disclosing information about the diagnosis to others (e.g., Hays et al., 1993; Mason et al., 1995; Stempel et al., 1995). Our focus is on the concerns of HIV-positive individuals about who to tell after they have learned about their diagnosis. We assume that there is a tension between the wish to reveal (e.g., to gain social support or medical information) and the need to conceal information about the diagnosis (e.g., fear of rejection, discrimination, or gossip). The need to balance the benefits and risks of self-disclosure makes it useful to examine, from the perspective of the HIV-positive individuals, their reasons for disclosing versus not disclosing the seropositive information to others.

A feature of our research is that participants provided data in open-ended interviews. We asked persons with HIV to recall the time shortly after they had learned about their seropositive diagnosis. In particular, we asked them to remember to whom they initially told information about the diagnosis as well as why they decided to inform this person. Similarly, we asked research participants to remember from whom they initially withheld information about the diagnosis as well as why they did not inform this person. These open-ended interviews (which also provided information about experiences with social support; see Chapter 5) lasted from 45 to 90 minutes. This procedure allowed us to explore in detail participants' reasons for disclosing or not disclosing information to various persons, relying on participants' own stories or accounts to generate the data.

Method

Research Participants

The sample consisted of 42 individuals with the HIV infection. The participants in the study were recruited from HIV/AIDS public service agencies in southeastern Virginia. There were 35 males and 7 females in the sample. The mean age of the participants was 34.02 years (standard deviation = 8.41). The participants were 28 African Americans, 10 whites, 1 Native American, 1 Hispanic, and 2 persons who were not identified ethnically. Most of the sample (36 of the 42 participants, or 85.71%) was not currently working, and 29 of the sample (69%) had earned less than $5,000 in the last 12-month period. A majority of the sample (26 participants, or 62%) had completed 12 or fewer grades of school. Twenty-four (57%) participants described themselves as homosexual, 9 (21%) as heterosexual, and 9 (21%) as bisexual.

Thirty-two individuals (76%) reported contracting HIV through sexual contact, 3 (7%) through drug injection, 3 (7%) through blood transfusion, and 4 (9.52%) said they did not know. The average CD4 cell count for the sample (based on participants' most recent reported results) was 290.8 (standard deviation = 272.9). See Chapter 5 for more details about the sample participating in the study.

Interview Procedure

Participants in the study were interviewed in private offices at an HIV/AIDS counseling organization. The focus of the interview was on the individual's experiences with social support provided by others (see Chapter 5) and the reasons for disclosing or not disclosing HIV-seropositive test results to others.

The self-disclosure segment of the interview was based on open-ended questions asking participants who they decided to inform or not inform when they learned about being HIV seropositive. The interviewer then asked participants to explain why they decided to disclose or not disclose the test results to these persons. The interviews were audiotaped and subsequently transcribed for coding. Each participant was paid $10.00 for the interview.

Data Analyses

The main focus of the data analysis was a content analysis of the reasons given by research participants for disclosing versus withholding information about the test results to specific persons. Participants' explanation for disclosure or nondisclosure could include more than one reason. One of the researchers developed a coding scheme based on an analysis of 10 randomly selected transcripts. The utility of this coding scheme was then verified by using it to code reasons for disclosure or nondisclosure on another 10 transcripts and then on the rest of the transcripts. Two other members of the research team also coded all the transcripts using this coding scheme, with a coding agreement of 92% for the reasons for disclosure and 94% for the reasons for nondisclosure. This level of coding agreement was considered satisfactory to conclude that the "reasons" were coded in a reliable manner. The coding of the reasons for disclosure or nondisclosure generated by the initial coder (D.L.) was used in the analyses reported in the Results section.

▧ Results

Reasons for Self-Disclosure of HIV-Positive Test Results

We coded 11 categories of reasons for disclosing about being HIV seropositive. These categories were

1. *Catharsis or self-expression* (5 of 114 reasons, 4.39%). The HIV-seropositive person hoped to feel better by releasing pent-up feelings. For instance, "I felt that I needed to get it [information about the HIV-positive diagnosis] out."

2. *Emotionally close and supportive* (42 of 114 reasons, 36.84%). This category focuses on the respondent's perceptions about the level of emotional closeness and support he or she has in a relationship with another person. It often involved feelings of closeness, caring, or trust for the other person, and that the other person would be understanding, consoling, concerned, and supportive. Illustrations of this category included "Because of the simple fact of me loving him [his partner]," and "We have always been close, and she has always been interested in everything that I have done."

3. *Forewarning* (14 of 114 reasons, 12.28%). The respondent wants to inform the other person so that the other person can prepare for what may happen in the future (including preparing for possible medical problems the respondent may have or that others might gossip and talk about the respondent's HIV-seropositive status). For example, "Because I wanted him to oversee his brother and sister when the time comes [that is, when the mother with HIV died]," and "In case something did happen [to me] I didn't want to wind up on her doorstep [that is, his mother's house], or to have somebody call her and say you know your son's got so and so."

4. *Loyalty* (6 of 114 reasons, 5.26%). The respondent feels loyal to family or friends and reveals the information because of that loyalty. For example, "Best friends tell best friends what is going on in their lives," and "I felt I'm their son, they have the right to know."

5. *Honesty* (8 of 114 reasons, 7.02%). The respondent shares the information because she or he wants to be honest or feels that informa-

tion about the HIV-positive diagnosis should not be hidden. For example, "We have never kept secrets and I wanted her to know why I am sick."

6. *Health concerns* (10 of 114 reasons, 8.77%). The respondent notifies someone, usually a present or past sexual partner, about their own HIV seropositivity so the other person will get tested or to indicate the importance of taking protective measures for safer sex. For example, "I was infected and there was a chance that he [the partner] could be infected . . . so he would need to go and find out if he was infected also," and "It was becoming physical and I felt that I had to let him [a boyfriend] know."

7. *Similar background* (6 of 114 reasons, 5.26%). Respondent reveals the information about the diagnosis to another person because they share a common background or experiences. The respondent may perceive that it is easier to share information with someone who sees the same physician or who is also HIV seropositive. For example, "Because he was dying of AIDS, he was in the same boat [as me]."

8. *Help* (8 out of 114 reasons, 7.02%). The respondent discloses information about the seropositive diagnosis because he or she needs information, material help, or some other type of tangible assistance. For example, "Because she [a friend] was in the health field and I figured she would be more knowledgeable [about HIV]. I thought she could be of help."

9. *Situational* (7 of 114 reasons, 6.14%). Someone else learns about the respondent's seropositive diagnosis as a result of a situation. There may have been others present in the room when the diagnosis was revealed to the respondent. For instance, "Because they [members of the family] are the ones who took me in [to the hospital] and the doctors told them."

10. *Educate* (7 of 114 reasons, 6.14%). The respondent discloses the HIV-positive diagnosis to educate others about the disease. For instance, "[I told him (a friend)] so that he could be aware of the fact that this illness is really serious and it can get anybody. You can look really healthy and still live with it and have it."

11. *Test other's reactions* (1 of 114 reasons, .88%). The respondent discloses information about the HIV diagnosis to see how the other person will react. "Because she [a sister] was so filled with hatred toward me and no compassion towards anyone else. It was almost like I have got to do something to make her feel something. Either she will hate me or she will love me for it."

Reasons for Nondisclosure of HIV-Positive Test Results

Respondents had also been asked to recall instances when they made the decision not to tell someone about being HIV seropositive after learning about the diagnosis. We coded seven categories of reasons for nondisclosure. These categories were

1. *Fear of rejection or of being treated differently* (30 of 91 reasons, 32.97%). The respondent felt that he or she would be treated differently if others knew about the HIV-positive diagnosis (e.g., fear of rejection, discrimination, or losing one's job). Illustrations of this category included "I kept it a secret from everyone because once you were diagnosed you were automatically plagued. All the overtures were negative. People didn't want to associate with you," and "I didn't want them [coworkers] to say don't touch her—that really scares me."

2. *Lack of understanding* (12 of 91 reasons, 13.19%). The respondent perceives that someone might show a lack of understanding, lack of support, or disappointment if they were told about the diagnosis. For example, "Certain things she [my aunt] doesn't understand and she doesn't try to understand," and "She [my sister] would throw it up in my face about being HIV or she would make jokes about it."

3. *Gossip* (19 of 91 reasons, 20.88%). The respondent fears that those told would spread the information to others if they knew about the diagnosis. For instance, "Once they [my sisters] find out they will call all over and tell all my family," and "If one person finds out then everybody will find out because people love to gossip."

4. *Protect other emotionally* (22 of 91 reasons, 24.18%). The respondent did not disclose the diagnosis because she or he was afraid that the information would upset the other person emotionally. There might

also have been concerns expressed about the possibility of other persons being stimatized if they were associated with a seropositive person. For instance, "It would scare her [my mother] and I did not want to scare her," and "I am afraid of them possibly getting the stigma about the legacy of it [HIV/AIDS], and [I] wouldn't want them to have anything to damage their confidence or esteem."

5. *Keep others from making sacrifices* (2 of 91 reasons, 2.20%). The respondent did not tell someone because the other person would have to make too great a sacrifice in caring for her or him. For instance, "I didn't want him [a son] to give up things he had going on in his life."

6. *Geographic separation* (2 of 91 reasons, 2.20%). The respondent cites geographic distance as a reason for not disclosing information about the HIV diagnosis to someone. For instance, "I don't want to give the information to them [friends] over the telephone and I have not been up there physically in person to see them."

7. *No way to tell* (4 of 91 reasons, 4.40%). The respondent may have felt that she or he wanted to tell someone about the diagnosis but they did not know how to or they were not prepared yet emotionally to talk about the disease to the other person. For instance, "I just didn't know how to tell him [partner], so I just hid from him most of the time and avoided him."

Reasons for Disclosing or Not Disclosing
HIV Test Results to Various Target Persons

Besides identifying the reasons given for disclosing versus not disclosing the HIV-positive diagnosis to others, we also wanted to know how the type of target person would affect reasons for disclosure or nondisclosure. Tables 8.1 and 8.2 present data (frequencies and percentages) about the impact of type of target (e.g., family, extended family, partner, ex-partner, etc.) on the use of various reasons for disclosure and nondisclosure, respectively.

Reasons for Disclosure to Targets. In general, family members (31 out of 114 times; 27.19%), friend (26 out of 114 times; 22.81%), and partner (19 out of 114 times; 16.67%) were mentioned most frequently in accounts of telling others about being HIV seropositive. Other target per-

TABLE 8.1   Reasons for Disclosure to Various Target Persons

	Family Member	Extended Family Member	Partner	Ex-partner	Friend	Acquaintance	Roommate	Coworker/ Supervisor	Health Professional	Public	Miscellaneous	Total
Catharsis		1 (11.11)		1 (16.66)	2 (7.69)			1 (33.33)				5 (4.39)
Emotionally close/ supportive	10 (32.26)	6 (66.67)	5 (26.32)	1 (16.66)	18 (69.23)		1 (25.00)		1 (20.00)			42 (36.84)
Forewarning	10 (32.26)						2 (50.00)	2 (66.67)				14 (12.28)
Loyalty	4 (12.90)			1 (16.66)	1 (3.85)							6 (5.26)
Honesty	1 (3.23)		4 (21.05)		2 (7.69)						1 (100.00)	8 (7.02)
Health concerns			7 (36.84)	3 (50.00)								10 (8.77)
Similar background			1 (5.26)		1 (3.85)	4 (80.00)						6 (5.26)
Help	1 (3.23)	1 (11.11)			1 (3.85)	1 (20.00)			4 (80.00)			8 (7.02)
Situation	4 (12.90)		2 (10.53)				1 (25.00)					7 (6.14)
Educate		1 (11.11)			1 (3.85)					5 (100.00)		7 (6.14)
Test other's reactions	1 (3.23)											1 (.88)
Total	31 (27.19)	9 (7.89)	19 (16.67)	6 (5.26)	26 (22.81)	5 (4.39)	4 (3.51)	3 (2.63)	5 (4.39)	5 (4.39)	1 (0.88)	114

NOTE: Each column presents the frequency of times that reasons for disclosure were associated with a certain type of target person. The percentage of times that a specific reason for disclosure was associated with a target person is shown in parentheses.

TABLE 8.2   Reasons for Nondisclosure to Various Target Persons

	Family Member	Extended Family Member	Partner	Ex-partner	Friend	Acquaintance	Roommate	Coworker/ Supervisor	Health Professional	Public	Miscellaneous	Total
Rejection/being treated differently	9 (23.08)	2 (25.00)	5 (62.50)	1 (33.33)	5 (33.33)	1 (20.00)		6 (60.00)			1 (50.00)	30 (32.97)
Lack of understanding	5 (12.82)	4 (50.00)				1 (20.00)		1 (10.00)	1 (100.00)			12 (13.19)
Gossip	5 (12.82)			1 (33.33)	7 (46.67)	2 (40.00)		3 (30.00)			1 (50.00)	19 (20.88)
Protect other emotionally	16 (41.03)	2 (25.00)	1 (12.50)	1 (33.33)	1 (6.67)	1 (20.00)						22 (24.18)
Keep other from making sacrifices	1 (2.57)		1 (12.50)									2 (2.20)
Geographic separation	1 (2.57)				1 (6.67)							2 (2.20)
No way to tell	2 (5.13)		1 (12.50)		1 (6.67)							4 (4.40)
Total	39 (42.86)	8 (8.79)	8 (8.79)	3 (3.30)	15 (16.48)	5 (5.49)		10 (10.99)	1 (1.10)		2 (2.20)	91

NOTE: Each column presents the frequency of times that reasons for nondisclosure were associated with a specific type of target person. The percentage of times that a specific reason for nondisclosure was associated with a target person is shown in parentheses.

persons (including extended family members, ex-partner, acquaintance, roommate, coworker or supervisor, professional, and public) were mentioned less frequently in personal accounts of notifying others about the seropositive diagnosis (see Table 8.1).

The most frequently cited reasons for disclosure to a family member were to get emotional support (32.26%) and to give forewarning (32.26%) about being HIV positive. In the case of extended family (such as cousins, uncles and aunts, or in-laws) the most frequently cited reason for disclosure was to get emotional support and understanding (66.67%). Thus, immediate and extended family members are likely to be disclosed to because the HIV-positive individual feels emotionally close to and supported by these persons, though giving forewarning about being HIV positive (i.e., to anticipate future problems such as the threat of gossip or health problems) was also a consideration in the decision to disclose to family members. Examining the column for friend as target of disclosure, it is interesting to note that emotional support was also a major reason for disclosure. Forewarning was never mentioned as a reason for disclosing to a friend.

When we examine the reasons given for disclosure to a partner, health concerns associated with sexual behavior were a major consideration. The health concerns category focused on telling the partner because he or she needed to be tested or the couple needed to practice safer sex. Another important reason for disclosure to the partner was because the respondent obtained emotional closeness and support in the relationship (21.05%). Also, honesty (21.05%) was cited as a reason for disclosure to a partner. The need for honesty as a reason for disclosure was not mentioned often with other target persons. When an ex-partner was mentioned as a disclosure target, it was usually for health concern reasons (i.e., this person might need to be tested for the HIV infection).

Acquaintances were mentioned several times as disclosure targets, usually because these persons were perceived as having shared similar backgrounds or experiences with the respondent. For instance, the respondent might report that they were both HIV positive or they were both gay men. Roommates were mentioned just a few times, and the reasons for disclosure to them were split among forewarning, emotional support, and the situation.

A coworker or supervisor was infrequently mentioned as a disclosure target, but forewarning was used as a reason 2 of the 3 times. A professional was notified about the diagnosis usually to elicit help (espe-cially information about the HIV infection and/or medications). The "public" was mentioned a few times as a disclosure target, but the only reason cited was to educate others about HIV infection and the AIDS epidemic.

Reasons for Nondisclosure to Targets. Family members were men-tioned most often (39 out of 91 times; 39%) in accounts of nondisclo-sure, followed by a friend (15 of 91 times; 16.48%) and coworker or supervisor (10 of 91 times or 10.99%). A roommate, professional, or "public" were rarely mentioned in personal accounts of withholding in-formation about the diagnosis from others (see Table 8.2).

The most frequently cited reasons for nondisclosure to a family member were to protect other emotionally (41.03%), fear of rejection or being treated differently (23.08%), lack of understanding (12.82%), and concern about gossip (12.82%). In nondisclosure to members of one's extended family, fears about lack of understanding (50%) and re-jection or being treated differently (25%) were mentioned as reasons for nondisclosure along with desire to protect the other emotionally (25%).

In reasons for nondisclosure to a partner, concern about rejection or being treated differently was mentioned most frequently (62.50%). In nondisclosure to a friend, concerns about rejection or being treated dif-ferently (33.33%) and gossip (46.67%) were often cited. For a coworker or supervisor, concern about rejection or being treated differently (60%) and gossip (30%) were usually mentioned in deciding to withhold infor-mation about the diagnosis from these persons.

Ex-partner, acquaintance, or health professional were not men-tioned frequently in accounts of nondisclosure about the diagnosis. When they were mentioned, reasons for nondisclosure to these targets cited concerns with rejection or being treated differently, lack of under-standing, and gossip.

■ Discussion

The present research illustrates how HIV-positive individuals con-sider the benefits and risks of disclosing versus concealing information about the diagnosis. Weighing the reasons for and against notifying others, HIV-positive individuals select whom they will tell as well as whom they will not tell about the diagnosis.

Having an emotionally close and/or supportive relationship (particularly with a friend, partner, family, or extended family member) was the major reason cited for disclosure to another person. The emotionally close/supportive reason emphasizes the socially mediated, personal benefit that may occur from self-disclosure about the HIV diagnosis: The recipient of the disclosure is expected to react with love, acceptance, and support. There were at least two other reasons for disclosure (although not mentioned frequently) that also represented socially mediated, personal benefits that are expected to derive from self-disclosure (disclosing to someone because of similar backgrounds and a desire for help). It might be expected that someone with similar experiences might be able to provide useful feedback on how to cope with the disease and, more directly, that disclosure about one's HIV status in the context of asking for help might lead to tangible assistance (e.g., useful medical advice or financial support).

Another benefit that was cited occasionally as a reason for self-disclosure was catharsis or releasing pent-up feelings about the disease. The reactions of the other person did not matter; however, disclosure allowed the person to vent feelings of rage, anger, anxiety, or fear associated with having contracted the disease.

We have noted the personal benefits that might occur from disclosing information about the diagnosis to others, including obtaining emotional support and help, talking with someone who has similar experiences, and catharsis. However, there are other reasons for disclosure that may not necessarily reflect personal concerns but emphasize a concern for another person or for a relationship with someone. For instance, an "other focus" was often involved in disclosures that were based on health concerns (the other person, usually a partner, should be tested for the HIV infection), desire to educate (the public should be informed about HIV), and forewarning (the others, usually immediate family members, will be forewarned so they can anticipate dealing with the discloser's future health-related problems and to forestall gossip). A "relationship focus," on the other hand, was involved in disclosures that were based on loyalty (usually to a family member; for instance, a perceived obligation to tell the other person) or out of a desire to have an honest and open relationship with someone (usually a relationship partner).

A concern about personal risks to self was the basis of some reasons for concealing information about the diagnosis from someone. These concerns included risks of rejection or being treated differently (usually a concern expressed about family members, partner, friend, or coworker or supervisor), others' lack of understanding (usually expressed about a family member or an extended family member), and gossip (a concern usually expressed about a friend). Interestingly, an other focus was also often involved in reasons for not disclosing to someone, based on a desire to protect the other person (usually a family member, parents especially) from being hurt or to keep the other person from having to make sacrifices.

We have presented evidence for a wide variety of reasons for disclosure and nondisclosure of the HIV diagnosis to others based on the self-, other-, or relationship-focused benefits or risks that the respondents had to address. The results are consistent with the view that HIV-seropositive persons weigh the benefits and risks of notifying others in their selection of whom to tell about the seropositive diagnosis.

Recalling the target persons cited in reasons for disclosure and nondisclosure, it is worth noting that family members (including parents and siblings) were mentioned frequently. These results indicate that family and friends may be perceived as sources of emotional support (especially friends) as well as persons to whom we may feel a sense of loyalty and obligation to forewarn about our personal difficulties (especially relatives from our family of origin). Nevertheless, family members and friends may also be perceived as sources of nonsupport who might be likely to reject us or treat us differently, show a lack of understanding, or gossip if they knew about the seropositive diagnosis. Thus, family members and friends may be viewed as persons who may or may not be told about the diagnosis, mirroring the mixed perceptions that individuals (including someone with the HIV infection) may have about significant others.

Although personal (self) concerns influenced many reasons for nondisclosure, the desire to protect someone (especially family members) from being upset also affected respondents' decisions not to disclose to others. Thus, a concern for others (despite one's own personal difficulties) may be a factor in the decision to refrain from talking to someone about the HIV infection. The desire to protect others' happiness (by not wanting to upset or worry them) is a frequent theme in reasons provided by individuals about why they do not disclose their HIV seropositive status to others in many studies (see, e.g., Hays, 1993; Mason et al., 1995).

A relationship partner was often cited as a disclosure target (because of perceived emotional closeness, support, health concerns, and having an honest relationship) but was also mentioned several times in the context of reasons for nondisclosure. Some respondents feared that they might be rejected or treated differently by their partner if they told the partner about their seropositive status. This concern is also cited in the results of other studies where seropositive individuals may not tell a new (or sometimes a long-term) partner about their positive test results for fear of scaring away or losing the partner.

Implications

Individuals experience considerable stress after learning that they are HIV positive. Notifying others about the diagnosis may play a helpful role in coping with the disease. But, as Hays et al. (1993) have noted, "disclosure of one's HIV seropositivity to significant others is a double-edged sword. It may open up the opportunity to receive social support. However, it may also lead to added stress, due to stigmatization, discrimination and disruption of personal relationships" (p. 425). The results of our research demonstrate that individuals seek to reduce the risks of self-disclosure (including the risks of being rejected themselves or being perceived to place unreasonable emotional or material demands on others) and enhance the benefits of disclosure (including obtaining emotional support and fulfilling relationship goals of loyalty and honesty) by selecting those to whom they will disclose information about the diagnosis. Selecting those who will have access to information about the HIV diagnosis (which is a form of privacy regulation) helps in resolving the tension between the need to share information about the diagnosis and also helps to preserve a sense of privacy and control over who has access to the information.

Several words of caution are necessary about our results.

We asked individuals to recall to whom they disclosed or from whom they concealed information about the diagnosis shortly after they had learned of their HIV seropositive status. The lists of reasons are fairly comprehensive, but the importance of reasons for and against disclosing information to significant others may vary based on the length of time since learning about the diagnosis or on the stage of the infection (e.g., Hays et al., 1993). For instance, members of one's family of origin may perhaps be told during a symptomatic or AIDS-diagnosed stage, compared to an asymptomatic stage, to forewarn them about health problems. As individuals integrate their seropositive status into their self-concept and feel less concerned about the reactions of others, certain reasons for not disclosing (e.g., gossip) may become trivial concerns.

It is difficult with the present research to draw conclusions about the impact of various demographic factors (e.g., sexual orientation, racial or ethnic background) on the types of reasons generated for disclosure or nondisclosure as well as on the type of target for disclosure or nondisclosure. The advantage of the intensive interviews was to provide data on the various reasons for telling others (or not telling others) about the diagnosis. Nevertheless, future research should focus on the impact of various cultural and economic backgrounds on decision making about disclosure. For instance, HIV-positive, gay men who are open to others about their sexual orientation may be less concerned about gossip than, say, HIV-positive gay men who have not talked about their sexual orientation to others (e.g., Mason et al., 1995). After learning themselves about the diagnosis, individuals who feel close to their families of origin may be more likely to disclose to family members out of a sense of loyalty or their own sense of closeness to them. People who are financially secure or well educated may be less concerned about their job security and, hence, may be more willing to disclose their seropositive status to, say, coworkers or a supervisor than would those who are financially precarious or poorly educated.

In summary, there may be many advantages and risks to disclosing one's HIV seropositivity to others. Our research indicates that HIV-positive persons consider the benefits and risks to themselves and others of talking about the diagnosis. Consistent with our idea of a privacy regulation model of disclosure, HIV-positive individuals weigh the pros and cons of disclosing information about the diagnosis to significant others and then select whom to inform.

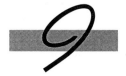

Factors Influencing Relationship Quality of HIV-Serodiscordant Heterosexual Couples

JAN MOORE
JANET SAUL
Centers for Disease Control and Prevention

NANCY VanDEVANTER
Columbia University

CHERYL A. KENNEDY
UMDNJ–New Jersey Medical School

LINDA M. LESONDAK
Georgia State University

THOMAS R. O'BRIEN
Viral Epidemiology Branch–National Cancer Institute

▧ Background

Research on chronic illness has substantiated that health problems are major stressors that can impair psychological functioning (Anderson, Anderson, & deProsse, 1989a; Leiber, Plumb, Gerstenzang, & Holland, 1976; Manne & Zautra, 1990; Revenson & Felton, 1989; Steele, Finkelstein, & Finkelstein, 1976; Woods, Haberman, & Packard, 1993). The human immunodeficiency virus (HIV) presents infected persons with a particularly stressful set of circumstances. First, HIV infection has a long, varied, and difficult course. For more than half of the people infected, the time from infection to the development of an AIDS-defining illness is more than 10 years (Rosenberg, Biggar, & Goedert, 1994). Increased access to HIV testing has resulted in more persons knowing their diagnosis early in the course of the disease. Consequently, many HIV-infected persons cope for years with the prospect and eventually the reality of a serious, debilitating illness that carries substantial social stigma. With the development of new treatments, HIV-infected persons are living longer and healthier lives. Despite these improvements in quantity and quality of life, HIV-infected persons must deal with the varied and unpredictable course of their disease and complicated treatment regimens that require great investments of time, energy, and money. The myriad stresses associated with HIV have been shown to greatly tax the emotional and psychological resources of infected persons. Emotional reactions such as grief, sadness, and fear; psychological difficulties including anxiety and depression; and social dysfunction including isolation and disrupted relationships have been widely documented as common responses to the burden imposed by HIV infection (Chesney & Folkman, 1994; Dew, Ragni, & Nimorwicz, 1990; Jacobsen, Perry, & Hirsch, 1990; Kamenga et al., 1990; King, 1989; Moore, Solomon, Schoenbaum, Schuman, & Boland, 1996; Moulton, Stempel, Bacchetti, Temoshok, & Moos, 1991; Ostrow et al., 1989; Peterson, Folkman, & Bakeman, 1996).

Like other serious illnesses, HIV infection affects the well-being not only of the infected individual but also uninfected persons intimately involved with him or her. For example, studies have documented distress in spouses and intimate partners, children, family members, and other caregivers resulting from the stress related to living with and caring for an HIV-infected person (Kamenga et al., 1990; Lippmann, James, & Frierson, 1993; Semple et al., 1993). Findings from studies of other serious health problems, including cancer, diabetes, and arthritis, have corroborated the effects of illness on the well partner (Leiber et al., 1976; Wellisch, Jamison, & Pasnau, 1978; Woods et al., 1993) and have demonstrated that, in some cases, well partners or spouses have more difficulty adjusting to illness than do ill persons (Coyne, Ellard, & Smith, 1990; Ekberg, Griffith, & Foxall, 1986; Flor, Turk, & Rudy, 1987; Wright, 1991).

Given the psychological consequences that health problems have on both the ill individual and on those intimately involved with him or her, it is not surprising that the functioning and quality of intimate relationships are also affected. A wide range of studies have shown that health problems may have a deleterious effect on the quality of close personal relationships (Anderson, Anderson, & deProsse, 1989b; Coyne & Smith, 1991; Elliot, Trief, & Stein, 1986; Gove, Hughes, & Style, 1983; Lewis, Woods, Hough, & Bensley, 1989; Manne & Zautra, 1990; Pratt, Schmall, Wright, & Cleland, 1985; Primomo, Yates, & Woods, 1990; Revenson, 1994; Wellisch et al., 1978; Woods et al., 1993). Although few data have been reported on relationships between HIV-infected persons and their partners, it is likely that this disease also affects relationships. In addition to the stresses that any serious illness place on a relationship, HIV infection requires that couples confront (a) the stigma associated with the disease and the potential social consequences of disclosure to friends, family, employers, health care providers, and so on; (b) decisions about changing sexual behavior to protect the uninfected couple member (if the partner is uninfected); and (c) in some cases, the HIV risk behaviors of the infected member that may have been unknown to the partner. Given the many challenges faced by couples coping with HIV, severe effects on relationship intimacy and communication would not be unexpected.

The present chapter examines factors that affect relationship quality among couples coping with HIV infection in one of its members. The literature on chronic disease and relationship quality suggests that some relationships deteriorate (Booth & Johnson, 1994; Klimes et al., 1992; Lewis et al., 1989; Peterson, 1979), some improve (Klimes et al., 1992; Leiber et al., 1976; Lichtman & Taylor, 1986), and some are unaffected by the illness of one member (Anderson et al., 1989a; Badger, 1990, 1992; Klimes et al., 1992; Leiber et al., 1976). A number of factors have been shown to influence which outcome couples will experience; however, two of the most important variables are severity of or degree of disability imposed by the illness and the psychological adjustment of individual couple members. This chapter examines the effects of stage of HIV disease and two measures of individual adjustment, depression and coping, on the relationships of persons dealing with HIV infection, an area that has received little attention in the literature. Data are presented from a study of HIV-infected persons and their partners that allow for examination of (a) the differential effects of disease on the ill individual and the well partner, (b) differences in functioning of couples in which the man is the HIV-infected couple member (referred to as male-infected couples) and those in which the woman is infected (referred to as female-infected couples), and (c) the influence of one couple member's adjustment on perceptions of the relationship by the other couple member.

Although different aspects of relationship quality have been examined in various studies (e.g., marital adjustment, satisfaction, intimacy, communication, sexual problems, conflicts), in the present analyses, two measures of relationship quality, intimacy and comfort communicating with the partner, are examined because of their potential relevance to couples dealing with HIV disease. Intimacy, the level of affection, trust, and cohesiveness within a relationship (Prager, 1995) may be particularly difficult to maintain for couples facing HIV as they attempt to alter sexual behavior to prevent transmission to the uninfected member, deal with risk behaviors of the infected member, and prepare for the eventual decline in health of the ill member. Thus, intimacy may be a sensitive measure of relationship quality for HIV-infected persons and their partners.

Communication is also a difficult area for couples dealing with HIV. Clinical observations and research have demonstrated that open, direct, and sensitive communication is critical to couples' successful adaptation to chronic disease (Helgeson, 1991; Rolland, 1994). The present study examines comfort communicating with the partner about HIV. Couples may avoid communicating about HIV because it is likely to raise painful issues for them. The need to plan for disclosure to friends and family, change sexual behavior, and make important health care decisions, however, requires extensive communication between couple members. Couples who have trouble communicating about the sensitive subject of HIV may have difficulty maintaining a quality relationship.

The present chapter examines these relationship issues among heterosexual couples in which one person is HIV infected and the other is uninfected (i.e., HIV-serodiscordant couples). Persons in heterosexual relationships are an increasingly large part of the HIV epidemic. Trends in AIDS cases reported to the Centers for Disease Control and Prevention (CDC) indicate that although cases among men who have sex with men are decreasing, the number of heterosexual persons with AIDS is increasing. For example, the proportion of adult and adolescent AIDS cases attributed to heterosexual transmission increased from 3% during the period from 1981 to 1987 to 10% during the period from 1993 to 1995 (CDC, 1995a). In addition, the proportion of AIDS cases due to injection drug use among heterosexual men increased from 20% of adult and adolescent cases in 1989 to 24% in 1995. AIDS cases attributable to sexual and injection drug use risk among men who have sex with men decreased from 71% in 1989 to 57% in 1995 (CDC, 1991, 1992, 1993, 1994, 1995a). If the present trend continues, more heterosexual persons are likely to become infected with HIV through either injection drug use or sexual contact, and the number of heterosexual couples coping with HIV/AIDS will thus continue to rise.

▓ The Sample

HIV-infected individuals and their uninfected heterosexual partners were recruited into a prospective study examining (a) rates of HIV transmission in heterosexual couples, (b) the biological and behavioral factors related to transmission, and (c) the effect of HIV on individual couple members and their relationship. Couples were recruited in New York City, San Francisco, and Newark, New Jersey via several sources, including HIV clinics, non-HIV medical clinics, HIV counseling and testing sites, private health care providers, public advertisements, other research studies, blood banks, and word of mouth. Data from participants in San Francisco were not included in the following analyses because some data were not collected at this site. Couples were eligible for the study if the uninfected partner had no reported risk for HIV other than sex with his or her infected partner and if the couple was sexually active during the 6 months prior to enrollment.

At the New York and New Jersey sites, 303 heterosexual HIV-serodiscordant couples were enrolled in the study; in 70% of the couples it was the male partner who was infected and in 30% it was the female partner. Because the study was designed primarily to examine the rates and causes of transmission, not all persons enrolled participated in the psychosocial component of the study, and only couples in which both partners completed the psychosocial component were examined in the present analyses. The present analyses were conducted on a sample of 197 HIV-serodiscordant heterosexual couples. Approximately half of the participants (52%) in this sample were white, 26% were Latino, and 22% were African American. Most had at least a high school education (81%) and reported a household income of more than $20,000 (70%). The median length of the couples' relationships was 5.3 years. The average time since diagnosis for the HIV-infected person was 33 months, and 17% had been diagnosed with AIDS. For 62% of the HIV-infected individuals, the probable route of infection was their own injection drug use, whereas for 35.5% the probable route of infection was sexual contact. The remaining 2.5% were infected through blood transfusion or through an undetermined route.

Male-infected couples were similar to female-infected couples with respect to race and ethnicity, length of time since the infected person was diagnosed with HIV, and level of HIV symptomatology. Members of female-infected couples were more likely to have a high school education (80%) than individuals in male-infected couples (65%), whereas the male-infected couples had been together for a longer period of time ($M = 2.5$ years) than the female-infected couples ($M = 2.2$ years). Injection drug use was the probable route of HIV infection for a higher percentage of HIV-infected men (73%) than women (37%).

Couples were followed every 6 months, at which time participants completed an interview on medical and sexual history, a physical examination, and a self-administered psychosocial questionnaire. Couple members completed interviews and self-administered questionnaires separately; the partner was not present during data collection. The two questionnaires included measures of sociodemographic characteristics, sexual behavior and condom use in the past 6 months, HIV-related communication, relationship characteristics, and psychological functioning. A more detailed description of scales and variables used in the current analyses may be found in the following sections. Only cross-sectional data collected at the baseline interview were used in the present analyses.

The remaining part of this chapter is divided into two major sections. The first section reviews the literature on the impact of severity or stage of illness on relationship quality and presents data on the influence of stage of HIV disease on intimacy and communication among HIV-serodiscordant couples. The second section examines the influence of psychological adjustment of individual couple members (i.e., depression, coping) on intimacy and communication within the relationship. Together these two sections offer a look at the factors affecting the functioning of heterosexual couples dealing with HIV infection.

▨ Stage of Disease and Relationship Quality

A diagnosis of HIV means that the infected individual will develop a serious and often fatal illness. However, if the diagnosis is early enough, there may be little impact on the health of the infected individual for an extended, although somewhat unpredictable, amount of time (Chesney & Folkman, 1994; Lifson, Hessol, & Rutherford, 1992; Moss & Bacchetti, 1989; Smith & Moore, 1996). Even though there may be little early physical dysfunction, receiving an HIV diagnosis is a traumatic event that often causes initial psychological distress. Most research has shown that persons typically adjust to an HIV diagnosis and resume normal functioning (Rabkin, Williams, Neugebauer, Remien, & Goetz, 1990); however, individual adjustment again declines with the onset of HIV-related symptoms and an AIDS diagnosis (Chesney & Folkman, 1994; Folkman, Chesney, Pollack, & Coates, 1993; Ostrow et al., 1989). Pakenham, Dadds, and Terry (1994) report that stage of HIV disease is the strongest predictor of psychosocial adjustment among HIV-infected gay men (i.e., the more advanced their illness, the lower their adjustment).

Besides affecting the adjustment and well-being of the infected person, stage of HIV disease has implications for the person's partner and the couple's intimate relationship. Research on diseases other than HIV has shown that more severe illness and higher levels of illness demands (i.e., more symptoms, declines in functioning, changes in roles) are related to lower levels of adjustment in the well partner and lower ratings of relationship quality (Anderson et al., 1989b; Lichtman & Taylor, 1986; Lewis et al., 1989; Peterson, 1979; Woods et al., 1993). As disease progresses, couples faced with HIV experience many of the same problems that couples dealing with other illnesses experience (e.g., increased physical disability, potential financial hardship, caregiving needs), but also some unique challenges, such as an increased need to disclose to friends and family as the infected person becomes sicker or concern about increased infectiousness. Thus, as HIV disease worsens, couple members are likely to experience significantly more burden and distress and may therefore have more difficulty maintaining their relationship. In the present analyses, the effect of stage of illness (defined by level of HIV-related symptomatology) is examined as it affects both intimacy and communication in the relationship.

Most studies examining couples' relationship quality have been unable to disentangle the effects of disease status (i.e., ill vs. well couple member) and gender because these factors are often confounded (e.g., male cardiovascular patients, female breast cancer patients). The design of the present study, however, allows for the examination of the impact of HIV status and gender because both male and female HIV-infected persons and their uninfected partners were assessed. The literature on adjustment to chronic disease suggests that well partners report lower relationship quality more often than ill partners (Booth & Johnson, 1994; Flor et al., 1987; Wright, 1991). Well partners frequently experience greater burden than ill partners; they often become caregivers to the ill partner and must assume greater responsibility for household duties and child care (Ekberg et al., 1986; Lichtman, Taylor, & Wood, 1987). These additional burdens may influence perceptions of the relationship with the ill partner. As with other diseases, well partners in HIV-serodiscordant couples are faced with the practical demands of the illness, such as caregiving and increased responsibility; however, they must also deal with additional emotional stressors. For example, HIV-uninfected couple members may experience a diminished sense of trust in their partner if they were not previously aware of their partner's risk for HIV. Also, HIV brings with it the possibility of infection for the uninfected partner, perhaps making sexual closeness unappealing. HIV- uninfected partners, faced with a potential decrease in trust and sexual closeness and increased pain brought on by death and dying issues, may distance themselves from the relationship. We hypothesize, therefore, that HIV-uninfected partners will report lower levels of relationship quality than infected couple members.

In addition to examining differences in ill and well partners, the design of the present study allows for the exploration of the differential effect of the disease on men and women. Gender differences in adjustment to disease have been reported in the literature; women tend to experience higher levels of depression and anxiety when adjusting to their own or their partner's chronic illness (Badger, 1992; Klimes et al., 1992). In addition, women frequently assume higher levels of caregiving burden than men that may add to their dissatisfaction in the relationship (Barusch & Spaid, 1989; Pakenham, Dadds, & Terry, 1995). In the present analyses, women were expected to express this negative view of the relationship by reporting lower levels of intimacy than their male partners. Conversely, it was hypothesized that women would report more ease with HIV communication. Communication research has demonstrated that women engage in more self-disclosure than men and are more likely to talk about personal aspects of their lives (Deaux, Wrightsman, Sigelman, & Sundstrom, 1988). In the present context, women were expected to express greater comfort than men in discussing the very sensitive topic of HIV.

In addition to the independent effects of stage of illness, HIV status, and gender, the present study examined the interactions of these variables. Although no specific hypotheses were made regarding the interactions, it was anticipated that differences between men and women might depend on which couple member was infected.

Method

Analyses

Because men and women's scores on the dependent variables were significantly correlated ($r = .47$, $p < .0001$ for intimacy; $r = .33$, $p < .0001$ for HIV communication), data were analyzed at the couple level (Kenny, 1988). A mixed design analysis of variance (ANOVA) with two between-couple variables, stage of illness and couple type (i.e., male vs. female infected), and one within-couple variable (gender) was conducted for the outcomes of intimacy and comfort with communication.

Measures

Stage of illness was a between-couple variable consisting of three levels (1 = AIDS; 2 = symptomatic but not diagnosed with AIDS; 3 = asymptomatic); the value for the couple was determined by the stage of illness of the HIV-infected partner. Couples were also divided into two couple types for the second between-couple variable: 1 = male-infected couples in which the man was the infected couple member and 2 = female-infected couples in which the woman was the infected couple member. Gender of the individual was a within-couple variable because each couple had both a male and a female member. The interaction of gender and couple type allowed for examination of HIV status of the individual (e.g., men in male-infected couples and men in female-infected couples could be compared).

Two measures of relationship quality were examined: intimacy and comfort with HIV-related communication with the partner. Intimacy was measured by an index of 6 items (Cronbach's alpha = .81) adapted from the emotional intimacy and intellectual intimacy subscales of the Personal Assessment of Intimacy in Relationships Scale (PAIR) developed by Schaefer and Olson (1981). Responses on the intimacy items were scored on a 5-point scale from *not at all* to *a great deal.* Examples of items on the intimacy scale included "My partner listens to me when I need someone to talk to" and "I often feel distant from my partner." Four items constructed by the investigators were summed to create an index of comfort with HIV-related communication within the study couple (Cronbach's alpha = .68). Items in this index included "Do you feel free to discuss HIV/AIDS with your partner?" (scored on a 5-point scale from *never* to *always*) and "How willing is your partner to talk to you about safe sex?" (scored on a 4-point scale from *very unwilling* to *very willing*).

Results

Intimacy

Scores on the two dependent variables (i.e., intimacy and HIV communication) were significantly correlated in this sample ($r = .40$, $p < .0001$). There were no significant main effects for stage of illness, couple type, or gender on ratings of intimacy. However, intimacy ratings were affected by a marginally significant interaction of gender of the infected person and stage of illness (see Table 9.1), $F(2, 183) = 2.51$, $p < .08$. Both men and women in female-infected couples reported higher levels of intimacy than members of male-infected couples, but only when the infected couple member had HIV-related symptoms, $F(1, 83) = 6.97, p < .01$. This difference in ratings of intimacy between female-infected and male-infected couples did not occur if the infected partner was asymptomatic or had been diagnosed with AIDS.

Communication

There was a significant main effect for gender when predicting comfort with HIV communication; men felt more comfortable communicating with their partners about HIV than women regardless of their HIV status or the stage of illness of the infected person, $F(1, 188) = 5.99$,

TABLE 9.1   Mean Rating of Relationship Intimacy and HIV-Related
Communication by Gender of the Infected Couple
Member and Stage of Illness

	Relationship Intimacy		
	Asymptomatic	*Symptomatic*	*AIDS*
Male-infected couples			
M	2.94[a]	2.72[a]	2.94[a]
SD	.70	.78	.51
n	48	58	26
Female-infected couples			
M	2.96[a]	3.16[b]	2.75[a]
SD	.78	.55	.79
n	23	27	7

	HIV-Related Communication		
	Asymptomatic	*Symptomatic*	*AIDS*
Male-infected couples			
M	2.88[a]	2.70[a]	2.86[a]
SD	.44	.58	.60
n	48	61	26
Female-infected couples			
M	2.89[a]	3.03[b]	2.66[a]
SD	.53	.48	.54
n	24	27	8

NOTE: Means in the same column that do not share the same superscript differ at $p < .05$.

$p < .02$. In addition, HIV-related communication was influenced by a marginally significant interaction of gender of the infected person and stage of illness, $F(2, 188) = 2.91$, $p < .06$. Consistent with findings on intimacy, both male and female members of female-infected couples reported more ease communicating about HIV than members of male-infected couples when the infected couple member had HIV-related symptoms, $F(1, 86) = 6.59$, $p < .01$. This influence of couple type on ease of communication was not seen among couples in which the infected person was asymptomatic or had been diagnosed with AIDS.

Discussion

The influence of stage of illness, couple type, and gender on relationship quality of HIV serodiscordant couples is complex. There was one significant main effect: gender. Men were more comfortable communicating about HIV with their partners than were women, regardless of which couple member was HIV infected. This effect was not hypothesized and seems counter-intuitive, given literature on communication showing that women engage in higher levels of verbal interaction than men in their close relationships (Deaux et al., 1988). However, in the present study we examined comfort communicating with the partner rather than amount of actual communication that occurs in the couple. Perceived openness of the partner to communication may be an important determinant of the other partner's comfort approaching HIV-related issues with him or her. Thus, a woman's greater proclivity for and openness to communication may result in her male partner feeling more permission than the woman to broaching this sensitive topic. An alternative explanation is that women are themselves uncomfortable talking about HIV. Women in couples faced with illness have been found to experience more depression and anxiety than men (Badger, 1992; Klimes et al., 1992). This negative psychological state may lead to less desire to communicate about a topic that is the source of their distress. Given the importance of communication for couples dealing with HIV, future research should examine gender differences in openness to discussions about HIV and responsiveness to communication attempts by the partner and how this affects not only the quality of the relationship but ability to negotiate and implement sexual behavior change.

Although the predicted main effects for stage of illness and couple type were not found, a marginally significant interaction was found between these two variables when predicting both intimacy and communication. Both men and women in female-infected as compared with those in male-infected couples reported higher levels of intimacy and comfort with communication only when the infected couple member was symptomatic but not yet developing AIDS. These higher levels were not present when the infected person was asymptomatic or had been diagnosed with AIDS. Several explanations can be offered for this complex pattern of results. First, the onset of symptoms is likely to signify declining health for persons in couples dealing with HIV. The threat of a decline in health could cause couple members to focus on their relationship and the significance of this event for the integrity and continuity of the relationship. Male and female couples may differ in their response to this threat, with members of female-infected couples moving closer and those in male-infected couples moving apart. Rolland's (1994) therapeutic work with couples facing illness offers an explanation for this pattern. He observed that, as a relationship focuses more on caregiving (as is the case when the ill member becomes sicker), couple members begin to interact more like parent and child, and adult intimacy is lost. When men are the caregivers, they are more likely to hire someone to assist with the caregiving role (e.g., housekeeper, nurse), whereas women attempt to add this caregiving role to those they are already fulfilling. Research supporting Rolland's observations has shown that women with illness are less likely to rely on the primary caregiver, usually the spouse, than are men and are more likely to use formal health services (Lorenson, 1985; Westbrook & Viney, 1983). Because men in female-infected couples may have sought outside help to assist with caregiving more than women in male-infected couples, this may allow female-infected couples to maintain a more intimate adult relationship.

An alternative explanation for the stage-of-illness-by-couple-type interaction is that the male-infected and female-infected couples in this sample differed from one another on dimensions that could affect relationship quality. For example, men who develop relationships with infected women may be much more different from other men than women who develop relationships with infected men are different from other women. Another explanation is that, in this sample, HIV-infected men were more likely to be intravenous drug users than HIV-infected women. The relationship quality of couples with a history of intravenous drug use (IDU) may differ from that of other couples. Unfortunately, we were unable to control for or stratify on drug use because of the low number of HIV-infected women with a history of IDU ($n = 22$).

The overrepresentation of persons with a history of IDU in male-infected couples could result in differences in relationship quality of male- and female-infected couples. The relation between couple type and relationship quality, however, was present only when the infected person was symptomatic. Thus, differences in proportion of drug users in male- and female-infected couples does not fully explain the finding. If, however, couples in which one person has a history of IDU have a particularly difficult time adjusting to the onset of symptoms, the couple-type-by-stage-of-illness interaction would be found. This pattern of results, which was only marginally significant in the present study, needs to be replicated in future research to substantiate that when faced with declining health, couples in which the woman is the ill partner are better able to maintain a quality relationship than couples in which the man is the affected couple member. Longitudinal data would allow for the examination of differences in adjustment of these two couple types as HIV disease progresses.

▓ Depression, Coping, and Relationship Quality

Research has shown that an important determinant of relationship quality for couples dealing with illness is the ability of individuals in that relationship to adjust to stress. Greater adaptability and resilience of individual couple members have been associated with better outcomes for the relationship, including greater marital satisfaction and intimacy and less discord (Booth & Johnson, 1994; Lewis et al., 1989; Woods et al., 1993). Two common indicators of individual adjustment, depression and coping, have been linked to relationship quality of couples with an ill member and are examined in the present analyses for couples dealing with HIV.

Depression is a frequent response to chronic illness by both the ill individual and the well partner, and an emerging literature has shown that depression in one or both couple members affects marital or relationship quality. Depression is frequently characterized by withdrawal from close contact and reduced interactions with others, and thus depression in the self or partner is likely to interfere with feelings of closeness in the relationship and desire for further interaction with the partner. In a large national sample of married persons, decrements in health were related to marital quality, primarily through the depressive behavior of the ill individual (Booth & Johnson, 1994). In a study of hemodialysis patients and their spouses, higher levels of depressive symptoms in the spouse were related to greater marital discord in the relationship (Finkelstein, Finkelstein, & Steele, 1976; Steele et al., 1976). Clinical reports and case studies have linked breast cancer to higher levels of depression in the spouse and to problems with marital adjustment (Maguire et al., 1978). In the present analyses, both self and partner's depressive mood are used to predict couple members' ratings of relationship quality and are expected to result in lower ratings of the relationship by both couple members.

The extent to which one couple member's depressive mood affects perceptions of the relationship may depend on whether the depressed person is the well or the ill partner. The literature on individual adjustment and relationship quality of couples dealing with chronic illness reports inconsistent findings about which (ill or well) partner's mood is most important for determining the quality of the relationship (Booth & Johnson, 1994; Finkelstein et al., 1976). Because the well partner is typically responsible for maintaining the functioning of the household and the well-being of its members, depression in the well partner may have a greater impact on the relationship than depression in the ill partner. Additionally, in the case of HIV disease, the infected person may feel responsible for the stress produced by his or her illness and thus may be particularly attuned to the emotional state of the uninfected partner. For example, an HIV-infected man whose female partner is depressed may feel less comfortable bringing up issues related to HIV than an uninfected man, particularly if he thinks his HIV is the source of her distress. In the current analyses, the uninfected partner's depression was expected to be a more important determinant of relationship quality than depression in the infected partner.

Data were analyzed separately for male and female couple members to examine gender differences in the influence of self and partner's adjustment on ratings of relationship quality. Data from studies of couples dealing with chronic illness suggest that women's depression may be more important than men's depression in determining how well the relationship functions (Fitting, Rabins, Lucas, & Eastham, 1986; Kotchick, Forehand, Armistead, Klein, & Wierson, 1996; Manne & Zautra, 1990) because women are often responsible for many of the day-to-day functions of a household and the emotional well-being of its members. In the present study, we also anticipated that depression in the woman would be more important for men's perceptions of the relationship than men's depression would be for women.

Coping strategies of individual couple members have also been linked to relationship quality of couples dealing with illness. Coping has been defined as the "cognitive and behavioral efforts to master, reduce, or tolerate the internal and/or external demands that are created by a stressful transaction" (Folkman, 1984, p. 843). Although coping responses have been classified along a number of dimensions, two broad groups are often distinguished: (a) avoidant strategies by which individuals distract attention from a stressor or deny its effect, thereby reducing its emotional impact, and (b) active strategies by which individuals directly affect the stressor by either actively changing the problem or cognitively changing the way the stressor is perceived (Billings & Moos, 1981; Cronkite & Moos, 1984; Folkman & Lazarus, 1980).

Avoidant coping strategies have typically been associated with poor outcomes for persons experiencing chronic illnesses (Berghuis & Stanton, 1994; Cronkite & Moos, 1984) and specifically for persons infected with HIV (Klein, Forehand, Armistead, & Wierson, 1994; Lichtman et al., 1987; Namir et al., 1987; Nicholson & Long, 1990; Pakenham et al., 1995; Wolf et al., 1991). Poor general psychological adjustment, depressive symptoms, and relationship problems have been linked to an avoidant coping style (Berghuis & Stanton, 1994; Bloom & Speigel, 1984; Causey & Dubow, 1992; Cronkite & Moos, 1984; Holahan & Moos, 1987; Manne & Zautra, 1989; Nicholson & Long, 1990; Vitaliano, Katon, Maiuro, & Russo, 1989). Active coping strategies have been less consistently associated with psychological outcomes in the literature. When associations are found, however, active strategies are linked to positive outcomes such as optimism, a sense of well-being, lower rates of depressive symptoms, and fewer marital difficulties (Berghuis & Stanton, 1994; Braithwaite, 1990; Brashares & Catanzaro, 1994; Namir et al., 1987; Pratt et al., 1985; Revenson & Felton, 1989; Vitaliano et al., 1989). In the HIV literature, active coping has been linked to enhanced mood and higher levels of self-esteem (Namir et al., 1987; Wolf et al., 1991).

A small but emerging literature has shown that coping strategies affect not only one's own well-being but that of close others as well. Manne and Zautra (1990), for example, found that the use of avoidant coping strategies by chronically ill women was related to poor psychological adjustment in their husbands. Klein et al. (1994) reported that among couples in which the man was hemophilic and in some cases HIV infected, the avoidant coping strategies of one couple member were related to depressive mood in the other member. The woman's use of avoidant coping, however, exerted a greater influence on the man's depression than the man's coping influenced the woman's depressive symptoms. In a study of adjustment to failed attempts at artificial insemination among infertile couples, Berghuis and Stanton (1994) found that men became more depressed if their female partners had high levels of avoidant coping, whereas women were less depressed if their partner used high levels of positive reframing and problem-focused coping. Although coping strategies of couple members are typically correlated, these studies demonstrate that one partner's coping exerts an independent influence on the psychological functioning of the other couple member.

In the current study, self and partner's use of active and avoidant coping were used to predict intimacy and comfort with HIV-related communication in the relationship. Hypotheses were straightforward for ratings of comfort with HIV-related communication: Men and women who use avoidant coping to deal with concerns about HIV are likely to feel uncomfortable discussing HIV-related topics with their partner, and those who adopt more active strategies are likely to feel more comfortable. Similarly, avoidant coping by one couple member is likely to cause the partner some discomfort in initiating discussions about HIV-related issues.

Hypotheses for the effect of coping on ratings of intimacy are less obvious. Self or partner's use of avoidant coping may restrict openness in the relationship and thus reduce the extent to which couple members feel intimate. On the other hand, persons who employ an avoidant coping style may actually perceive their relationships as more intimate. HIV may be perceived as a threat to the stability and continuity of a relationship, particularly for the HIV-infected member. Persons who use avoidant coping tend to deal with threats by distracting attention from or denying the effects of the stressor. Reporting enhanced intimacy in a relationship may help the avoidant individual draw attention from or deny fears and anxieties about the effect of HIV on one's relationship. Thus, avoidant coping may either decrease or increase ratings of relationship intimacy. Hypotheses for active coping are also not immediately obvious for the intimacy outcome. Individuals who use active coping are, however, typically oriented to solving problems and thus are likely to be problem solvers in their relationships also. If this is the case, then active coping by the self or partner is likely to produce healthier, better-functioning relationships and, therefore, higher reports of intimacy.

HIV status and its interaction with coping strategies of the self and partner are also examined in the following analyses. As with depression, the importance of self or partner coping may depend on who is the HIV-infected couple member. The literature from other chronic diseases has shown that coping of both the ill and well partners can influence relationship outcomes (Berghuis & Stanton, 1994; Klein et al., 1994; Manne & Zautra, 1990), and partners were thus expected to influence one another regardless of their HIV status. However, as with depression, the well (i.e., uninfected) couple member's coping may be more important for relationship outcomes than the HIV-infected person's coping.

The effect of coping on ratings of relationship quality were examined separately for male and female couple members, thereby allowing for examination of gender differences in the influence of self and partner's coping on perceptions of the relationship. Data suggesting that the woman's adjustment is more important than the man's in determining how well the family and relationship function suggest that the woman's coping may be more important for relationship quality than the man's coping (Klein et al., 1994). On the other hand, women have been shown to be more empathic than men (Lang-Takac & Osterweil, 1992; Trobst, Collins, & Embree, 1994) and may thus be more attuned to the coping strategies of their partner than are men. If this is the case, men's coping strategies will be more important for determining women's views of their relationship than women's strategies will be for men.

Method

Analyses

Hierarchical multiple regression analyses were performed to determine the unique contribution of self and partner's adjustment (i.e., depressive mood or active and avoidant coping) on ratings of relationship quality. HIV status and the measure of adjustment for the self were entered in the first block and measures of adjustment of the partner were entered in the second block. Given that adjustment scores of couple members are often correlated and were for depression in the present analyses ($r = .35$ for depression; $r = -.01$ for avoidant coping; $r = .01$ for active coping), hierarchical regression allowed for the determination of the independent influence of partner's adjustment on relationship ratings above that contributed by adjustment of the self. Finally, the interaction of HIV status and adjustment scores for the self and the partner was entered in the third block.

Measures

The Center for Epidemiologic Studies Depression Scale (CES-D) was used to measure depressive mood or symptomatology for all study participants (Radloff, 1977). Participants were asked 20 questions about how they felt during the previous week, such as "I felt lonely" and "I had crying spells." A 4-point response scale was used (0 = *rarely or none of the time* to 3 = *most or all of the time*) and an index was formed by summing the items (Cronbach's alpha = .91).

Participants were asked how often they had used various strategies over the past 6 months to deal with their concerns about HIV/AIDS. These strategies were adapted from standard coping scales to be specific and relevant to HIV-related concerns. Two scales were constructed using factor analysis: (a) active coping (Cronbach's alpha = .72), which included items measuring behavioral actions and cognitive reconstruction, and (b) avoidant coping (Cronbach's alpha = .74), which measured both denial and distraction.

Results

Depression and Relationship Quality

Women's Ratings. As in previous research, women who had higher scores on depressive mood reported less intimacy and comfort communicating with their partner than those with lower ratings of depressive mood (see Table 9.2). Male partner's depressive mood, however, did not affect women's ratings of intimacy or women's comfort with communication. A main effect for the woman's HIV status was also found: Women who were HIV infected reported greater intimacy in their relationship than did uninfected women. HIV status did not interact with own or partner's depression, however, to affect ratings of relationship quality.

Men's Ratings. Men with higher levels of depressive mood also reported less intimacy and comfort with communication in their relationship (see Table 9.3). This effect, however, was qualified by an interaction of depressive mood and HIV status such that the man's depressive mood was related to ratings of relationship intimacy and comfort with communication for HIV-uninfected men but not for infected men.

TABLE 9.2 Summary of Hierarchical Multiple Regressions Predicting Women's Intimacy and Comfort With HIV Communication

	Intimacy			HIV Communication		
	Block 1	Block 2	Block 3	Block 1	Block 2	Block 3
Variables	β	β	β	β	β	β
Women's HIV status	.15*	.14*	.10	.06	.06	.13
Women's depression	-.31***	-.29***	-.33***	-.31***	-.30***	-.29***
Men's depression		-.06	-.03		-.04	-.01
Women's HIV × women's depression			.10			-.02
Women's HIV × men's depression			-.05			-.07
R^2	.12***	.13***	.13***	.10***	.10***	.10***
ΔR^2		.01	.00		.00	.00

NOTE: ΔR^2 = increase in variance accounted for each block of variables.
*$p < .05$; **$p < .01$; ***$p < .001$.

Men's ratings of comfort with HIV communication were affected by their partner's level of depressive mood: The more depressive the mood reported by the female partner, the less comfort with HIV communication reported by the man. An interaction effect of HIV status and depression, however, indicated that the partner's depression affected the man's comfort communicating with his partner only if he was HIV infected. For uninfected men, comfort with communication was unrelated to their female partner's depression.

Coping and Relationship Quality

Women's Ratings. As in the analyses using depression as a predictor, a main effect was found for the woman's HIV status on her ratings of intimacy: HIV-infected women reported more intimacy in their relationship than uninfected women (see Table 9.4). This effect, however, was qualified by an interaction of the woman's own use of avoidant coping and her HIV status. HIV-infected women who were high on avoidant coping reported greater intimacy in their relationships than low-avoidant HIV-infected women. There were no other significant effects of coping on intimacy. In terms of comfort with HIV communication, women who had higher scores on avoidant coping were less comfortable communicating with their partner than less-avoidant women. An interaction effect for active coping and HIV status was found with higher scores on active coping associated with greater comfort communicating for HIV-infected women but not for HIV-uninfected women.

The male partner's use of avoidant and active coping were related to the woman's comfort communicating with him: The less avoidant and the more active coping he reported, the more comfort the woman reported communicating with him about HIV.

Men's Ratings. For men, both intimacy and comfort with communication were affected only by their own use of avoidant coping (Table 9.5). The more avoidant coping reported by the man, the less he reported feeling intimate and comfortable communicating with his partner. The female partner's coping did not affect men's ratings of relationship quality.

TABLE 9.3 Summary of Hierarchical Multiple Regressions Predicting Men's Intimacy and Comfort With HIV Communication

	Intimacy			HIV Communication		
Variables	Block 1 β	Block 2 b	Block 3 β	Block 1 β	Block 2 β	Block 3 β
Men's HIV status	.04	.03	-.24	-.07	-.08	-.14
Men's depression	-.37***	-.32***	-.62***	-.25***	-.18*	-.50***
Women's depression		-.12	-.18		-.20**	.01
Men's HIV × men's depression			.44**			.50**
Men's HIV × women's depression			.08			-.33*
R^2	.13***	.15***	.18***	.08***	.11***	.16***
ΔR^2		.02	.03*		.03**	.05**

NOTE: ΔR^2 = increase in variance accounted for each block of variables.
*$p < .05$; **$p < .01$; ***$p < .001$.

TABLE 9.4 Summary of Hierarchical Multiple Regressions Predicting Women's Intimacy and Comfort With HIV Communication

	Intimacy			HIV Communication		
	Block 1	Block 2	Block 3	Block 1	Block 2	Block 3
Variables	β	β	β	β	β	β
Women's HIV status	.15*	.14	-.35	.09	.10	-.61*
Women's active coping	.10	.09	.06	.09	.06	-.08
Women's avoidant coping	-.14	-.12	-.25*	-.17*	-.15*	-.17
Men's active coping		.05	.03		.21*	.14
Men's avoidant coping		-.10	-.11		-.20*	-.23*
HIV × women's active coping			.09			.55*
HIV × women's avoidant coping			.44*			.03
HIV × men's active coping			.09			.17
HIV × men's avoidant coping			-.03			.06
R^2	.05*	.05	.08	.04	.08*	.12**
ΔR^2		.00	.03			.04*

NOTE: ΔR^2 = increase in variance accounted for each block of variables.
*$p < .05$; **$p < .01$; ***$p < .001$.

187

TABLE 9.5 Summary of Hierarchical Multiple Regressions Predicting Men's Intimacy and Comfort With HIV Communication

Variables	Intimacy			HIV Communication		
	Block 1 β	Block 2 β	Block 3 β	Block 1 β	Block 2 β	Block 3 β
Men's HIV status	.03	-.03	.29	-.05	-.05	.00
Men's active coping	.06	.06	.09	.13	.14	.03
Men's avoidant coping	-.20*	-.21*	-.24	-.27**	-.28**	-.27
Women's active coping		-.01	.03		.04	.17
Women's avoidant coping		.03	.13		.00	-.02
HIV × men's active coping			-.06			.24
HIV × men's avoidant coping			.04			-.01
HIV × women's active coping			-.08			-.24
HIV × women's avoidant coping			-.18			.03
R^2	.03	.03	.04	.06**	.07*	.08
ΔR^2	.03	.00	.01	.06**	.01	.01

NOTE: ΔR^2 = increase in variance accounted for each block of variables.
*$p < .05$; **$p < .01$; ***$p < .001$.

Discussion

As seen in research on other illnesses, adjustment of individual couple members was related to ratings of relationship quality. Depressive mood in the self was related to lower ratings of relationship quality for women and for HIV-uninfected men. Typically, the link between depression and relationship quality is thought to result from the depressed person's impaired ability to relate to and communicate with their partner, thereby producing relationship problems. Except for one condition in the present analyses (HIV-infected men's ratings of comfort with HIV communication), partner's depressed mood did not result in lower ratings of relationship quality by the other couple member, suggesting that partners do not share the depressed couple member's negative view of the relationship. Perhaps depression in the self results in a negative view of many aspects of one's life, including one's relationship, rather than causing "real" relationship problems. Depression has been shown to result in more negative, although in some cases more realistic, assessments (Alloy & Abramson, 1979). Lower ratings of relationship quality may merely reflect this bias among depressed persons. Longitudinal studies with more refined measures of relationship quality are needed to better understand the impact of the individual's adjustment on the ability of couples to thrive under the stress of illness.

Coping strategies, like depression, were also related to ratings of relationship quality, although the patterns of associations were not always consistent with predictions. As expected, both men and women who had high levels of avoidant coping indicated less comfort communicating with their partner about HIV. Additionally, women whose male partners reported high levels of avoidant coping indicated less comfort with HIV-related communications. This finding is particularly troublesome if discomfort with HIV-related communication results in diminished ability of the couple to work out the many issues related to HIV, including planning, negotiating, and implementing safer sex practices. If this is the case, use of avoidant coping by the self or partner could result in greater risk of HIV transmission. An avoidant coping style may also affect comfort with HIV-related activities beyond communication with the partner. For example, disclosing HIV status to friends and family; seeking support, advice, and medical attention; and participating in behavior change interventions may be particularly difficult for avoidant individuals because these activities force them to direct attention to the topic they are trying to avoid, HIV. Future research should examine the relation between use of avoidant coping and willingness to participate in interventions related to sexual behavior change, to seek medical attention, or to disclose HIV status. If persons who use an avoidant strategy have particular difficulty with these activities, ways to engage them without triggering avoidant coping would be essential for successful HIV-prevention activities (McKirnan, Ostrow, & Hope, 1996).

As we predicted, men who had high scores on avoidant coping rated their relationships as less intimate. Men who use avoidant coping to deal with the many stresses associated with HIV may find it particularly difficult to be intimate with the partner who has the potential to bring painful issues to their attention. By remaining closed to and distant from the relationship, the avoidant individual may feel some protection from the many difficult issues related to HIV and the partner. This strategy may also, however, cut him off from the potential support of the partner. Future research is needed to determine if consequences of an avoidant coping style include alienation and isolation from intimate social relations.

The pattern of association between avoidant coping and intimacy was not the same for women: HIV-infected women who used avoidant coping to deal with HIV rated their relationship as more intimate than less-avoidant HIV-infected women. Their avoidant coping, however, was not related to their male partner's perceiving greater intimacy in the relationship, suggesting that male partners do not share the avoidant woman's enhanced view of the relationship. HIV-infected women with uninfected partners may feel particularly vulnerable and have underlying doubts about the continuing support of their male partner. Women who deal with HIV through avoidance may enhance perceptions of intimacy in their relationships in an effort to deny or avoid anxieties and fears about the stability and continuity of the relationship.

Both depression and coping influenced partner's comfort with communication more than it affected intimacy ratings. These findings suggest that although the partner's adjustment may not affect general closeness in the relationship, couple members are able to detect when partners may have difficulty dealing with HIV, as would depressed persons and those coping with HIV through avoidance, and consequently feel uncomfortable initiating discussions about the topic. In these situations, the couple member who appears more fragile and unable to cope (i.e., the person who is depressed or is using avoidant coping) may actually control the couple's ability to have frank, open discussions about issues central to the functioning and well-being of the couple. Further research is needed to determine how couples in which one or both members experience individual adjustment problems change interaction patterns to protect those persons from difficult topics.

The data presented are cross-sectional, and thus the direction of causality between individual adjustment and relationship quality cannot be determined; individual adjustment difficulties could cause relationship problems, relationship problems could add to individual difficulties, or both could occur. Generally, the literature suggests reciprocal relations between individual adjustment and quality of marital or couple adjustment. In the present data, we have examined one segment of that reciprocal influence. Although other explanations are possible, our interpretations of the data are substantiated by a significant literature from longitudinal studies demonstrating the importance of individual adjustment for the quality of couples' relationships. The current data in addition to these previous studies suggest that interventions aimed at improving individual adjustment (e.g., teaching coping skills, alleviating depression through psychotherapeutic techniques or anti-depressant medication) may also affect the quality of intimate relationships of HIV-infected persons.

Summary

The data from these analyses suggest that the relationship quality of heterosexual couples dealing with HIV is influenced by a complex array of factors. First, the functioning of the couple may depend on whether the man or woman is the HIV-infected couple member. Second, ratings of the quality of the relationship differ for men and women. Third, perceptions of the relationship are influenced by the couple member's own psychological adjustment as well as the adjustment of his or her partner, although these effects are complex and sometimes depend on gender and HIV status. Finally, the same factors do not have an impact on all aspects of relationship functioning (i.e., communication and intimacy in the relationship).

These data offer a beginning understanding of the factors that influence couples' adaptation to HIV infection. Additional research is needed that (a) follows couples dealing with HIV to examine differences in the adaptation of male- and female-infected couples to the stresses presented at the different stages of HIV disease, (b) examines the mechanism by which the individual adjustment of couple members affects the functioning of the relationship, (c) examines the adaptations that couple members make to protect vulnerable members from potentially distressing topics and how these adaptations affect the functioning of the relationship, and (d) examines the ways that relationship problems (e.g., lack of intimacy or communication) affect the ability of couples dealing with HIV to react to and cope with challenges such as disclosure and sexual behavior change.

Public Disclosure of HIV
Psychosocial Considerations for Children

LORI S. WIENER
National Cancer Institute, Bethesda, MD
NANCY HEILMAN
Good Samaritan Hospital, Puyallup, WA
HAVEN B. BATTLES
National Cancer Institute, Bethesda, MD

The Centers for Disease Control and Prevention (CDC) (1997) currently estimate that there are 7,902 children (under 13 years old) with AIDS in America, and 2,953 cases of AIDS in adolescents (13 to 19 years old). As an increasing number of children who are born infected with human immunodeficiency virus (HIV) live to older ages, the question becomes more crucial of when and how to talk with them about their illness, as well as who else should be told about the diagnosis (Abrams & Nicholas,

AUTHORS' NOTE: We would like to thank the children and families at the Pediatric Branch of the National Cancer Institute who shared their time and expertise about disclosing their HIV diagnosis to the public. We would also like to acknowledge Tina Chernoff, John Daly, Naomi Lampert, Kristin Riekert, and Gayl Selkin-Gutman for their assistance in the collection of disclosure data and Lani Leary for her help in coding the interviews. Special thanks go to Dr. Philip Pizzo, Chief of the Pediatric Branch of the National Cancer Institute, for his generous support of this research.

193

1990; Lipson, 1993). In addition to the growing number of children infected with HIV, there are many thousands of children profoundly affected by the impact of HIV on a close family member—a mother, father, sibling, or other relative in the kinship network (Tasker, 1992). The CDC currently estimates that 1 in every 100 males and 1 in every 800 females are HIV infected (CDC, personal communication, May, 1995). Yet the initial reaction of many adults upon learning of their own or a family member's HIV diagnosis is that the diagnosis must be kept a closely guarded secret. Disclosure of either the parent's or the child's HIV diagnosis to a child is a controversial and emotionally laden issue. One reason that was frequently cited by parents and family members in our clinic[1] for not disclosing is the fear that the stigma of AIDS will have a negative impact on children and their families. At the other end of the spectrum are those families that choose to publicly disclose an HIV diagnosis. There are a number of reasons that a family may choose to go public with their child's diagnosis. However, the lack of literature in this area served as an impetus to conduct a study to directly examine the impact public disclosure has on the HIV-infected child and family. This chapter will examine the results and implications of this study.

HIV/AIDS and Stigma

AIDS has been labeled the most controversial disease in modern history (Powell-Cope & Brown, 1992). Because of society's misperception that one can only be infected through "socially unacceptable" behaviors such as homosexuality, drug use, and sexual promiscuity, HIV and AIDS are highly stigmatizing medical conditions. AIDS has been shown to elicit negative and fearful attitudes from high school students (Huszti, Clopton, & Mason, 1989), adults (Dawson, Cynamon, & Fitti, 1987), medical students and residents (Kelly, St. Lawrence, Smith, Hood, & Cook, 1987a, 1987b; Link, Feingold, Charap, Freeman, & Shelov, 1988), and physicians (Loewy, 1986). This stigmatization has led to social ostracism of people with HIV/AIDS. For a more comprehensive look at the stigmatization of HIV and AIDS, see Chapter 2.

Given the effects of stigma, it is not surprising that many parents are hesitant to disclose their own or their child's HIV diagnosis. Weiner, Perry, and Magnusson (1988) conducted an attributional analysis of reactions to stigma. They found that for stigma perceived as uncontrollable, such as blindness, Alzheimer's disease, cancer, heart disease, paraplegia, and Vietnam War syndrome, subjects responded with more pity, less anger, greater liking and more willingness to provide personal assistance and/or charitable donations. However, for stigma perceived as controllable, such as child abuse, drug addiction, obesity, and AIDS, subjects responded with more anger, less liking, little pity, and low judgments regarding willingness to provide personal assistance and/or charity. In the case of an HIV-infected child who has contracted the virus perinatally or through a transfusion, people may view him or her as blameless, and thus the child would receive more support from others. Going public with a child's diagnosis may be an attractive option.

By contrast, a study by Levin et al. (1995) surveyed the attitudes of neonatologists about the treatment of conditions unrelated to HIV for critically ill newborns at risk for HIV. A substantial proportion of the respondents in this study recommended less aggressive treatment for both HIV-positive infants and children of HIV-positive mothers who were only at risk for HIV. Such recommendations appeared to be associated with low estimates of the infants' potential quality of life. These results are illustrative of the potential pervasive and lasting effects of HIV-related attitudes.

Disclosure of a Stigmatizing Illness

For individuals with potentially stigmatizing conditions, the issue of disclosure may be of major concern. Limandri (1989), for instance, reported that individuals who perceived themselves as having a condition that society disapproves of or views with disgust (such as herpes or AIDS) may often attempt to conceal their condition—even from health care providers. Conditions under which disclosure is likely to occur include appropriate relationship level with receiver for revealing, appropriate situational context, appropriate comfort level with receiver, and favorable receiver characteristics such as trustworthiness and likability (Braithwaite, 1991; Petronio, Martin, & Littlefield, 1984). Disclosure also requires that the discloser be willing to be vulnerable enough to tell his or her secret. Once this happens, there is often a small revelation to "test the waters" by disclosing the secret to a stranger (Limandri). If this goes well, further disclosure often follows (Jourard, 1972; Yalom, 1985).

Clinical experience indicates that privacy appears to be an essential condition for disclosure of the diagnosis to the child in many families.

Many parents worry that their child(ren) would not be able to maintain the secret of his or her diagnosis. Just as Limandri (1989) described in a sample of three types of disclosers (HIV-infected individuals, victims of domestic abuse, and individuals with herpes), parents of HIV-infected children at the National Cancer Institute (NCI) often describe telling their child's diagnosis to a stranger whom they will never see again to help anticipate others' reactions. If this does not evoke a negative response, parents may then disclose their child's (or their own) diagnosis to those who are closer to them. Logic would suggest that if disclosure of the diagnosis to individuals who are close to the family goes well, the family will feel more comfortable engaging in further disclosures, which may then lead to voluntary public disclosure.

In order for unilateral disclosure to occur, the discloser must anticipate that he or she will benefit in some way that will outweigh the sense of exposure (Hays et al., 1993; also see Chapter 9). Hays et al. found that among a sample of HIV+, gay men, disclosure of one's diagnosis may have contributed to improved psychological well-being when the person being disclosed to responded in a helpful manner. The men in this study also indicated that the reasons they chose for not disclosing their diagnosis to others included not wanting to upset others, fear of discrimination, fear of disrupting relationships, feeling that others would have little to offer in the way of support, and desire to conceal one's homosexuality or mode of transmission. These reasons are similar to those observed in our clinic. Many parents of HIV-infected children at NCI describe trying to balance the pros and cons of disclosing the child's diagnosis both to the child and to the child's school. For many, the cons outweigh the pros, and, as a result, much tension remains about when to inform the child and others of the child's diagnosis. For others, the sheer relief of not having to keep a secret any longer, or the support that they anticipate receiving, may be enough to convince them to go public.

In Chapter 2, Leary and Schreindorfer discuss the concept of stigma avowal and describe a subgroup of persons with HIV who incorporate their disease as a positive basis of their social identity by publicly declaring their condition. Such individuals may choose to give public lectures or be active in AIDS-related causes. It is suggested by Leary and Downs (1995) that these individuals may receive positive social benefit from the HIV population, resulting in increased self-esteem. In their review of self-disclosure, Derlega et al. (1993) concluded that concealing any information that is threatening to the self is correlated with physical and emotional problems. On the other hand, Braithwaite (1991), when discussing results from her study of disclosure of personal information by disabled people to able-bodied people, suggested that disclosure may not always be advantageous for the disabled person. Simply meeting the emotional needs of the able-bodied person may be more effort than it is worth. Likewise, HIV-infected individuals (or their caregivers) may find it to be stressful to manage the emotional reactions of non-HIV-infected individuals when disclosing the diagnosis.

Effects of Secrecy on Self-Esteem and Personal Distress

Crocker and Major (1989) have argued that being stigmatized may protect one's self-esteem because negative feedback from others could be attributed to one's stigmatizing condition. Thus, if children were aware of their HIV diagnosis, they might then be able to protect themselves from negative interactions by attributing them to their serostatus. This follows from Crocker and Major's theory, but a more likely scenario may be that knowledge of one's diagnosis, particularly for those children who are public with their diagnosis, may offer children a sense of importance in that they may have the opportunity to educate others about the disease. Coopersmith (1967) found that children from 10 to 12 years old who have high self-esteem have a closer relationship with their mothers than do those children with low self-esteem. Thus, self-esteem may also be enhanced simply by knowing that one's parents have been honest. In this study, children's ratings of global self-worth are used as an outcome measure to examine whether or not disclosure is beneficial to the child.

Tasker (1992) reported that keeping an HIV diagnosis a secret often results in personal distress and loneliness. The energy required to maintain secrecy creates distrust and tension for everyone involved. Pearson (1981) suggested that keeping the diagnosis a secret can have a very negative impact on both parents and children. Both clinical experience at NCI and clinical accounts related by Tasker (1992) and Wiener and Septimus (1994) suggest that not being able to talk about the virus with others is one of the most difficult aspects of having a child who is HIV-infected. The stress associated with withholding the diagnosis is tremendous. Disclosing the child's diagnosis to important others appears to markedly relieve this stress. It is not clear whether disclosing the diagnosis to the public is equally, if not more, beneficial. For this reason, both depression and caregiver's social support satisfaction were assessed in the present study.

Emotional Impact of Public Life
and Media Coverage on Children

There has been little research on the emotional impact of public life on children. Most of the literature pertaining to the mass media and the AIDS epidemic focuses on the misrepresentation of people with AIDS by the media (Albert, 1989; Biddle, Conte, & Diamond, 1993), especially the homophobic or "heterocentric" view of HIV/AIDS by the media (Hallett & Cannella, 1994). Libow (1992) described her clinical observations of traumatized children and the news media. She wrote primarily about children who had been victims of natural disasters and were then picked up by the news media. Many of her observations still apply to the population of which we are speaking who, for the most part, have actively chosen to go public with their HIV diagnosis.

Libow (1992) noted that although it is conventional to obtain informed consent from parents in addition to assent from the child when involved in a research study, it is rarely obtained from children who are to be featured in the media. Even when it is obtained, it is rarely truly informed. Children, particularly young ones, are not likely to fully understand the ramifications of being featured, for example, on the evening news. One 9-year-old girl was horrified at the fact that her schoolmates had seen her on the news giving an interview in her pajamas. She had no concept of the reach of television into her friends' homes, nor did her parents have any idea of the child's inability to foresee this reality (Libow, 1992).

Changes in the Child's Perceived Identity

Children who had survived a school-bus kidnapping reported that they hated a monument in their town erected in their honor because it reminded them of the helplessness they felt during the kidnapping (Terr, 1983). Similarly, a child who becomes known as the "kid with AIDS" may grow tired of that identity and wish to be seen as a "normal" kid rather than as a sick one.

Children who have survived disasters are often portrayed as heroes because they have survived, rather than being recognized as children who may have lost a great deal such as their homes, friends, or family members (Libow, 1992). Children with HIV are often treated the same way. They are hailed as children of tremendous courage and strength and not recognized as children who are dealing with an often painful and frightening illness that may well have already claimed one or more of their family members.

How Publicity Affects Others

Libow (1992) talks about "poster children" or "mediagenic kids," children who are singled out to serve as a representative of many other child victims. These children are often socially skilled, attractive, and articulate. After being seen on television or in the newspaper, they are frequently bombarded with gifts and contributions from well-intentioned strangers who want to help. Children who have gone public with their diagnosis often have opportunities to meet celebrities and to travel to places to which they would not ordinarily have gone. These charitable acts are both helpful to the family and, at times, detrimental. One mother reported that her 13-year-old daughter said, while on a private tour of the White House, "I'm glad I have AIDS." When her mother questioned her on this statement, the girl responded that she would not have been able to do all these neat things if she had not had AIDS. This may seem like an unfortunate consequence of public attention, but perhaps it enables the child to effectively deal with his or her illness. In addition, many individuals, children and parents alike, indicate that the feeling of having educated or helped others is highly reinforcing.

By contrast, children who are not in the public light may feel hurt and confused as to why their tragedy is not being recognized. David, an 8-year-old HIV-infected boy at the NCI, asked, "Is his AIDS better than mine?" after seeing a "public child" in a television documentary who had what he thought was the same illness as his. Clinical experience has shown us that many HIV-infected children who are not public are often inspired by those who are in the public light. Many factors appear to be associated with one's desire to be public. These include an ability to be open about one's disease, the knowledge of who can be counted on for support, and the secondary effects of the media attention associated with publicity, such as material benefits.

▓ The National Cancer Institute HIV-Disclosure Study

The remainder of this chapter will summarize the findings of a study designed to examine the impact of public disclosure on HIV-infected children and their families. Specifically, findings pertaining to the decision-making process, the impact public disclosure has had on the child's family, satisfaction with one's social support, and the child's sense of self-worth will be reviewed as they pertain to the emotional impact publicity has on the child. Special attention is directed toward those children who had limited support prior to "going public" and the lifestyle changes that occurred afterwards. Interventions and strategies aimed at counseling families considering going public and helping to normalize the public child's life are discussed.

Method

Observations forming the clinical basis for this research were made during routine visits to NCI for medical treatment. Although it was clear that families who have used the mass media looked forward to their public appearances, children and parents often discussed these experiences in different terms. At times, staff became concerned that the patient may have been an unwilling participant or that the caregiver was motivated purely by secondary gains. As other families began considering media disclosure, they looked to staff to help guide their decision making based on the experiences of families already in the limelight. Therefore, as part of a larger study examining parents' styles of disclosing their own HIV diagnosis to their child(ren), as well as the child's own HIV positive (HIV+) diagnosis to the child, data were collected from the 18 families seen at the Pediatric Branch of the National Cancer Institute who have chosen to share their story with the media. To the authors' knowledge, this is the first systematic study of such "mass media" families, their motivations, and the general assessment of their experiences. For the purposes of this study, *being public* was defined as the experiences of HIV-infected children who had shared their name and diagnosis in the media (either TV or newspaper).

Participants

The Pediatric Branch of the National Cancer Institute offers treatment to HIV-infected children who meet criteria eligibility for a clinical trial. Since the program began in December, 1985, 475 children have been followed under our care. Our patient population originates from all over the United States and does portray a national cross-section. However, our sample represents resourceful families that have been able to enroll their children in a national research protocol. In addition, the majority of our families are Caucasian, and a greater percentage of children in the present study have been infected through a transfusion (45.7% for entire sample; 77.8% for "public" sample) than is representative of the pediatric AIDS population in the US (10.7%) (CDC, 1995b). This is not the average profile of a typical U.S. family dealing with a child who is HIV-infected.

Both primary caregivers and their school-age children who were enrolled in one of the HIV clinical protocols at the Pediatric Branch of the National Cancer Institute during the summer of 1994 were invited to participate in the study. Primary caregivers (foster or kinship families) who (a) had not had the child in their care when the diagnosis was disclosed or (b) had not had the child in their care for the past 6 months were not invited to participate in this study.

From 124 parent-child dyads who were selected and also agreed to participate in our study, 105 were retained in the final analysis (a response rate of 83%), and 18 families were identified as being "public." The gender and ethnicity composition of the public children were 14 males, 4 females; 15 Caucasians, 2 African Americans, and 1 Latino. Four of the public children had acquired HIV "vertically" (i.e., mother-to-child), 5 acquired it through a transfusion of contaminated blood, and 9 acquired the disease as a result of a hemophilia-related transfusion of coagulation factors. All 4 of the children who acquired HIV vertically were accompanied by their adoptive parents, and thus the words "parent" or "caregiver" in the following sections will refer to their adoptive parent. The other 14 children were accompanied by a biological parent. Children ranged in age from 9 to 21 years, with a mean age of 13.2 years and a standard deviation of 3.7 years. Of the 87 children who were "not public," 54 were male, 33 were female; 63 were Caucasian, 15 were African American, and 9 were Latino. Of these children, 52 had acquired HIV vertically, 18 through a blood transfusion, and 17 who were hemophiliacs had acquired HIV through a transfusion of coagulation factors. Age ranged from 5 to 19 years, with a mean of 10.3 years and a standard deviation of 3.6 years. The public children tended to be older (13.24 years) than those who were not public (10.54 years), but there was no significant difference in their ages.

Procedure

The purpose of the study was explained to each parent and informed consent (given by parents for both themselves and their child) was obtained. Caretakers were asked to complete the Beck Depression Inventory (Beck, 1967), the Arizona Social Support Interview Schedule (ASSIS; Barrera & Ainley, 1983), and the Family Environment Scale (FES; Moos & Moos, 1993). The Self-Perception Profile for Children (SPPC; Harter, 1985) was administered to children between the ages of 8 and 13 years; the Self Perception Profile for Adolescents (SPPA; Harter, 1988) was administered to children between the ages of 14 and 18 years. Children and caretakers were also questioned about their emotional reactions to public disclosure via a structured interview format.

Measures

Structured Interview. The interview of both the children and their caregivers (administered separately) was designed to examine the emotional reactions to public disclosure in the mass media. It included open-ended questions concerning what children and parents remembered about the time when they decided to go public, how they went public, how public they had been, whose decision it had been to go public, how the media had treated them, how their family and friends had reacted to the decision to go public, from whom they received the most and least support since going public, whether or not they would recommend public life for other families, and the best and worst things that had happened to the family since going public. Responses were hand recorded by the interviewer and then a quantitative analysis was completed by three separate raters to extract the major themes. Once the major themes were extracted and agreed on by the three raters, all responses were coded by one rater.

The Beck Depression Inventory (Beck, 1967). This 21-item, multiple-choice measure assesses the frequency of symptoms of depression. Each question has four choices (scored 0 to 3), with each successive choice indicating an increase in the severity of the symptom. Results from this instrument have been shown to correlate highly with clinician ratings of severity of depression, behavioral ratings of depression, and other self-report measures of depression (Rehm, 1977). Internal consistency for our sample was $\alpha = .89$.

Arizona Social Support Interview Schedule (Barrera & Ainley, 1983). This scale measures the various facets of social support by obtaining quantitative information on positive and negative social contacts. A slightly modified version of the ASSIS (Mitchell, 1989) was selected for this study and permits us to draw distinctions between social network members who are supportive versus those who are sources of conflict. The ASSIS yields five social support indices: total network size, unconflicted network size, conflicted network size, support satisfaction, and support need. Response format varies between the different support indices. The three network sizes are determined by summing the number of people indicated for each of the different types of networks. Unconflicted network size is measured by asking the subject questions such as who (first names or initials only) he or she would talk to about things that are very personal and private. Conflicted network size is measured by asking with whom the subject can expect to have negative interactions. Total network size is measured by summing the unconflicted and the conflicted networks, making sure to count each listed person only once. The support satisfaction and need scales are scored on a 3-point Likert-type scale. The support satisfaction subscale score is ascertained by asking subjects how many opportunities, ideally, they would have liked to have had to engage in each of the four unconflicted interactions in the last month (ranging from "it was just about right" to "I would have liked a lot more opportunities"). Support need is determined by asking subjects how much they felt they needed, for example, to talk about things that were very personal and private (ranging from *not at all* to *quite a bit*). Internal consistency for the social support indices ranged from α = .52 to α = .54.

Family Environment Scale (Moos & Moos, 1993). This measure comprises 10 nine-item, true-false subscales. These subscales are as follows: Cohesion, the degree of commitment, help, and support family members provide for one another; Expressiveness, the extent to which family members are encouraged to act openly and to express their feelings directly; Conflict, the amount of openly expressed anger, aggression, and conflict among family members; Independence, the extent to which family members are assertive, are self-sufficient, and make their own decisions; Achievement Orientation, the extent to which activities (such as school and work) are cast into an achievement-oriented or competitive framework; Intellectual-Cultural Orientation, the degree of interest in political, social, intellectual, and cultural activities; Active-Recreational Orientation, the extent of participation in social and recreational activities; Moral-Religious Emphasis, the degree of emphasis on ethical and religious issues and values; Organization, the degree of importance of clear organization and structure in planning family activities and responsibilities; and Control, the extent to which set rules and procedures are used to run family life. The possible range for all subscales of the FES is 0 to 9. Internal consistency ranged from α = .17 to α = .73 on the Family Environment subscales. Low internal consistency scores were found on the Independence (α = .26) and Control (α = .17) subscales, indicating that these subscales were not reliable measures for this sample. The remaining subscales all had internal consistencies of at least α = .53.

Self-Perception Profile for Children. This instrument measures the construct of self-perceived competence using a 4-point, forced choice, Likert-type scale ranging from "really not like me" to "really like me" (Harter, 1985). The child form (for ages 8 to 13 years) and adolescent form (Harter, 1988) share six subscales measuring self-perceptions of scholastic competence, social acceptance, athletic competence, physical appearance, behavioral conduct, and global self-worth. The adolescent form contains three additional subscales measuring self-perceptions of job competence, romantic appeal, and close friendship. The scale is standardized for children over the age of 8 years, is easy to administer, and takes approximately 10 to 15 min to complete. Internal consistency for the child form ranged from $\alpha = .54$ to $\alpha = .82$. Internal consistency for the adolescent form ranged from $\alpha = .22$ to $\alpha = .96$. The subscale with the lowest internal consistency was the job subscale, indicating that this subscale may not have been valid for our sample. All of the remaining subscales had internal consistencies of at least $\alpha = .59$.

Results

Themes Expressed by Children and Parents About Public Disclosure of HIV

The First Challenge: Deciding Whether to Go Public. Responses to the parent and child interviews are summarized in Table 10.1. All of the children and parents interviewed in our study who had gone public with the HIV diagnosis reported that the decision had been painstaking and difficult. One 12-year-old girl, who had recently completed a TV documentary, illustrated this point clearly when asked what one of her worst experiences was since learning of her own diagnosis. She replied, "making the decision to go public."

During the open-ended interview, children and parents were separately asked what helped them the most in making the decision to go public. About 50% of both children and caregivers reported that it was their desire to tell the truth and to not have to lie or deceive others. Seventeen percent of children reported being inspired by another child with HIV who had already gone public, and 20% of parents wanted to educate others. Slightly fewer than half of the parents and children reported that it was the child's decision to go public, 33% of children and 47% of parents reported that it was the parent's decision, and 17% of children and 7% of parents reported that it was the decision of both the parents and the child. Twenty-seven percent of parents reported feeling relieved after the first public disclosure took place.

Taking the Steps to Disclose Publicly. One third of both parent and child respondents reported that their first step in going public was to inform the child's school of the diagnosis. Twenty-two percent of children and 20% of parents reported telling a friend as their first step, and

TABLE 10.1   Child and Caregiver Responses to Structured Interviews
($n = 18$ dyads)

	Child (%)	Caregiver (%)
What helped you make the decision to go public?		
Desire to tell the truth/escape the secrecy	44	47
Wanted to educate others	5	20
Going public was not their decision	11	13
Inspired by another child with HIV	17[a]	
Have you ever been on a talk show?		
Yes	75	75
No	25	25
If you were on talk shows, did you feel the host really cared about you?		
Yes	61	47
Mixed feelings	22	33
No	0	0
Did you ever feel used?		
Yes	17	47
No	67	47
Who have you gotten the most support from?		
Family/friends	72[b]	33
Media (child)	11	
Public (parent)		7
Other parents or people living with AIDS	n/a[b]	27
Who have you gotten the least support from?		
Nobody	44	0
Community	28	20
Family	6	27
Do people treat you differently since going public?		
No difference	44	27
Receive more attention/view us as celebrities	22	33
People are nicer/more concerned	11	27
Has going public changed your relationships with your friends?		
No change	50	40
Better	39	40
Worse	0	0
Has going public changed your relationships with your family?		
No change	50	40
Better	33	53
Worse	0	0
If you could do it (go public) all over again, would you?		
Not sure	6	13
No	11	7
Yes	83	80

a. Questions whose values do not add up to 100 indicate that there were a number of responses that could not be meaningfully coded.
b. Some children gained support from other people living with AIDS, but they referred to these people as their "friends."

17% of children and 27% of parents reported their first step to be disclosing on television. Two thirds of both parents and children reported that their next (second) step was to be in a newspaper; approximately 10% reported going on TV next. Although only 22% of children and 20% of parents identified telling a friend their diagnosis as their first step in going public, 78% and 80% answered "yes" when asked if they told their close friends their diagnosis before going public. This disparity in responding is likely to be a function of perceptions of "going public." Many respondents may not have considered telling a close friend to be the beginning of the public disclosure process. When asked, in reference to telling their close friend, "How did that go?" 50% of children and 80% of parents indicated that telling the close friend had been a positive experience. Only 17% and 13% of children and parents, respectively, said it went poorly; the other 33% and 7% gave neutral answers.

The Media Experience. The nature of these families' HIV-related mass media exposure varied from being interviewed frequently by their local newspaper or radio host to participating in numerous national TV talk shows. For several of the children, being "on the road" to give lectures and TV interviews had become a way of life.

Subjects were asked how often they had appeared on TV shows and how they felt the host had treated them. One child said of his media experience, "Most of the media uses you, the other quarter becomes your friends. They'll do what they can to get a story." Although only 78% of children thought that their parents were keeping a scrapbook of their public appearances or articles, every parent who was interviewed reported keeping a scrapbook. Parents described feeling "very proud" of their child's accomplishments and said that keeping a scrapbook helped them "remember the positive parts of living with HIV." Families also reported that the scrapbooks would become a part of their child's legacy that they will hold on to and cherish forever.

The Impact Public Life Has on Relationships With Friends, Family, and Others. Children and their caregivers were asked who they had received the most and least support from since going public and how their relationships with family and friends had changed. These responses are summarized in Table 10.1. When asked how the other children in the family reacted to public life, about one third of both children and parents reported that the siblings felt jealous, left out, or were generally having a hard time with it. One parent said of her noninfected daughter, "Debbie feels left out, not important. She wants the attention, but when she gets it, she shies away from it. [She has] mixed feelings—[she's] happy for the attention, but sad because she feels like she is not a part of anything and nobody cares about her." One half of parents and only 6% of children reported that their siblings were supportive of the new life.

Would You Do It All Over Again . . . and How? When the children and parents were asked "if given the chance," would they go public all over again, 83% of the children and 80% of parents reported "yes," and 11% and 7% said "no." Forty-four percent of children and 40% of parents said that if they were to do it all over again, they would do it the same way, and 39% and 27% said they would do it differently, some indicating that they would do it sooner or that they wouldn't be as afraid of it. Only one parent and two children said they just wouldn't do it. Sixty-seven percent of children and 40% of parents would recommend with very few reservations that other families go public. Thirty-three percent of children and 60% of parents recommended it with strong reservations, saying that not everyone could handle public life and that they should wait until the time was right for them. When asked if they ever wished they could go back to just being themselves, not a "well-known" person living with AIDS, 61% of children and 47% of parents said "yes." Although it seemed in the answers that many respondents may have been referring to their wish not to be HIV-infected rather than not to be public, specific comments highlighted their ambivalent feelings regarding the attention they received. One 10-year-old girl illustrated this point well by stating "sometimes I kind of get sick of everyone saying 'hi' to me all the time . . . being so nice to me. People tell me 'you just get away with everything because you have HIV.' I don't think that's always true." Most other comments, however, reflected the following sentiment: "There are days you wish that you could go back to being private and not public with HIV." There was an existential flavor to some of the comments that reflected an ability to balance the negative and positive sides of a public life. "It is worth it if it will make it easier for the others to come" and "I would want to go back to a non-public life if life could be normal (whatever that is) but on the other hand I don't want to because the experiences we have endured in this lifetime both inward and outward are things I wouldn't give up for the world."

Social Consequences of Going Public. Fifty-six percent of the children reported that the best thing about going public was being able to do new things, meeting celebrities, and receiving gifts and money. Twenty-eight percent said the best thing was all the support they received, and 17% were happiest about not having to lie anymore. Forty percent of parents reported that the best thing about going public was the opportunity to educate others, 27% enjoyed the support they received, 13% reported a sense of freedom and happiness, and another 13% felt that either their child's physical or mental health had improved. One boy's mother said the following of her public experience: "I have had the opportunity to touch thousands of lives through love, experience and education that I would have never otherwise done. I also was able to utilize my audiences as my support system." Fifty-six percent said the worst thing about going public was the negative response they received from certain others. These responses ranged from being teased to a barber refusing to cut one boy's hair to one family's house being burned down for having three HIV-infected children in the home. Eleven percent of children disliked always being in the public eye and not being able to be a "normal kid." One child complained that "Everyone keeps an eye on me. Everyone knows me. I can't act like a regular kid. Everything I do gets a lot of attention. It's a constant reminder of my disease." However, 28% of the children could not identify a "worst thing" associated with going public. Twenty percent of parents felt that the worst thing about going public was their child's pain. For example, one mother reported that the worst thing she had to deal with was "the pain and heartache that my son has had to go through just to show the world that he was a person just like everyone else and that he had to use the press to be heard with his feelings." Thirteen percent of parents reported being contacted by "medical quacks" with miracle cures, another 13% were not pleased with the media, and another 13% mentioned the bad reaction from the public (e.g., house being burned down, other kids not being allowed to play with their kids). Twenty-seven percent did not identify anything as being their worst experience since going public.

Public Disclosure Versus Non-Public Disclosure

When comparing those children in the study who had disclosed their diagnosis publicly with those who had not, the two groups failed to differ on a number of variables, including CD4%, which was used as an indicator of disease severity. The CD4% is the percentage of total lymphocytes that are CD4 cells (as opposed to the absolute CD4, which is the actual number of CD4 cells). There were also no significant differences among parents on the Beck Depression Inventory (Beck, 1967), which measured parental depression. In fact, generally speaking, parents did not score in the clinically depressed range.[2] However, potentially interesting patterns were found in the areas of family environment, child's self- esteem, and parental social support. These findings are discussed below.

Profile of Family Environment in Public Families. A series of independent sample *t* tests were conducted comparing the children who were identified as being public with those who were not but were part of the larger study. A broad, general profile of family characteristics in the public group was suggested by the data. However, none of the findings pertaining to family environment attained statistical significance at the traditional .05 level and should therefore be interpreted with caution. When compared to families who declined to share their HIV diagnosis with the mass media, public families tended to be more expressive, report the presence of more family conflict, and rate themselves as being more satisfied with their social supports.

Families who had shared their diagnosis with the public tended to score higher ($M = 6.69$, $SD = .22$) than nonpublic families ($M = 6.03$, $SD = .04$) on the FES Expressiveness scale, although the difference in scores did not reach significance ($p = .14$). A high score on the FES Expressiveness scale suggests that family members are actively encouraged to act openly and to express feelings directly. This finding is corroborated by clinical observation, as the public families were inclined to be more verbally oriented and articulate in their day-to-day interactions with NCI staff. The FES Conflict scale was also somewhat higher (albeit not significant, $p = .12$) in public ($M = 3.85$, $SD = .29$) versus nonpublic families ($M = 3.15$, $SD = .04$), which suggests that anger, aggression, and conflict may be more openly expressed among members of families in the public eye. Results on other subscales of the FES failed to even approach statistical significance, indicating that the two groups did not differ on Cohesion, Independence, Achievement Orientation, Intellectual-Cultural Orientation, Active-Recreational Orientation, Moral-Religious Emphasis, Organization, or Control.

Social Support. The ASSIS Support Satisfaction scale yielded divergent response patterns between the two groups, with public families exhibiting a trend toward having more need for support ($p = .12$) and less satisfaction with perceived social supports ($p = .12$) than nonpublic families. Although we must be cautious in drawing conclusions from nonsignificant findings, these trends are surprising and unexpected, as the public families seem to have so many people who care about them and how the HIV-infected child is doing. Whether public families have a greater desire than nonpublic families for opportunities to interact with others about things that are personal may be worth examining in future research. It may be that the support being provided to the public families is coming from people they do not know well compared to people they have known for some time (celebrities or people who have heard their story through the media). It may also be that this finding is an artifact of the families in this group being more expressive in general. Another plausible explanation supported by clinical observation is that this need for more interpersonal interactions is secondary to the overall sense of isolation that is often expressed. Public families may experience this isolation on a different plane, especially if they come to be known as "The Family With AIDS." The other scales of the ASSIS (Unconflicted Network Size, Conflicted Network Size, and Total Network Size) failed to approach significance.

Child's Self-Esteem. Statistical significance was attained on four of the Harter Self-Perception Profile for Children subscales (for ages 8 to 13 years) but was not always in the expected direction. Children who were public with their HIV diagnosis tended to perceive themselves as being less scholastically competent ($p < .001$), being less socially competent ($p < .05$), having fewer positive physical attributes ($p < .01$), and having a lower global self-concept ($p < .01$) when compared to children who were not public. This was an especially puzzling finding in that the "public kids" tended to be among the best-known, well-liked children in the NCI clinic, and it was not unusual for other children to make attempts to interact with and emulate them. We were less surprised by the Scholastic scale being lower. Although we failed to collect data systematically on academic achievement, the public children were less likely to attend school regularly or be part of a regular classroom situation (32%, vs. 2% for nondisclosed group). In most cases, the parents chose to have their children tutored at home, sometimes as a means to accommodate a child with many social engagements or public appearances. For some children, the high level of skilled medical care necessitated a home-tutoring arrangement. Because we were unable to collect pre- and post-data, it is unknown whether lower self-esteem is a product of being in the public eye, or if lowered self-esteem existed before public disclosure. The decision to go public could be viewed as an attempt to deal with or bolster an inadequate self-concept. Data from the adolescent scales yielded no significant findings. This may have been primarily due to the extremely small number of adolescents ($N = 6$) who were identified as publicly disclosing their HIV-positive status. This small sample size affected the reliability of the analysis, preventing an adequate test of the effects of going public for the adolescents.

Implications for Future Research

The findings in this study must be considered preliminary and clearly require replication. Several limitations to the generalizability of the present findings need to be addressed. First, the sample of children who went public about their HIV-positive diagnosis was not entirely representative of the demographic profile of children living with HIV infection in this country. Of these 18 children, the majority were male, Caucasian, and acquired the disease through a transfusion of contaminated blood. None of the children were living with a biological parent who was also HIV infected. Perhaps public sympathy would not be as great for a family perceived as having infected their child. Second, given the small sample size, we could not examine the impact of variables such as age, ethnicity, culture, geographic location, or the effect of public disclosure on well siblings. Third, each of the children had been public for different lengths of time. A longitudinal design could have assessed individual and family changes that have taken place for several years after public disclosure. Baseline data on each child's self-esteem, social support, or family environment would have been useful, as these variables may have changed after the child went public. In addition, baseline data would have afforded the researchers the opportunity to obtain a profile of those children and families who do choose to use the media. For example, were certain characteristics such as the parent-child relationship, degree of emotional isolation, and/or quality of social support important variables for those families who chose to go public? It may also be useful to examine the child's and parents' personality factors, which may predict or coincide with those who choose public disclosure.

Fourth, it is well known that social support is an important moderator for reducing stress (Cobb, 1976; Cohen & Wills, 1985; Dean & Lin, 1977; Fullerton, McCarroll, Ursano, & Wright, 1992; House, Landis, & Umberson, 1988; Kessler & McLeod, 1985). The scale used to assess support (ASSIS) was designed to tap a more intimate support (e.g., family members, close friends) than the potential behavioral or mental health benefits of public support. A more effective measure for assessing a family's satisfaction with public support would be one that specifically taps the domain of public support.

Finally, we did not investigate how these children may have been strengthened or helped to become more resilient by their public experience. Several of the children seemed to use their speaking engagements and television interviews as an opportunity for mastery—allowing them to feel in control of their disease and its associated treatments and to feel proud of their ability to reach out and touch other lives. Future studies should focus on coping strategies and the effects of public exposure on adaptation.

This study was a first attempt at understanding the emotional reactions of public disclosure on HIV-infected children. The findings clearly underscore the need for future empirical studies addressing disclosure in general and disclosure to the media in particular.

Implications for Clinical Practice

It has been our experience that each family of an HIV-infected child eventually wrestles with the question of disclosure in some way. It may just be a question of who to tell among their close friends or who to tell at the child's school. For some this decision will entail mass media participation. When patients come to their clinician for direction and advice on this matter, we suggest the following guidelines be applied.

Both the child and parents should be invited to discuss their goal for publicly disclosing an HIV diagnosis. Who will benefit the most from public disclosure? This is an important question, as almost one third of the children we interviewed reported that it was their parents' decision, not their own, to go public. What do they hope for or fantasize about as an end result? Using the responses and experiences of the families presented in this chapter, it is sensible to determine if the child's and parents' goals are reasonable and appropriate. For instance, many parents have reported that they allowed their children to make public appearances because they believed such activities would help the children feel better about themselves. The data from this study suggest that an increase in the child's self-esteem is not a common outcome.

It is also recommended that the whole spectrum of going public be explored with the family. If the primary goal is to educate others about living with HIV disease, one alternative to full disclosure is to lecture or be featured on TV in another state or to use a fictitious name and avoid identifying photography. We believe such partial disclosure tactics are a good way to enter public life. Using this method, family members are able to get a sample of such experiences without putting their personal life and identity on the line. It also allows parents a more controllable way of seeing how their child reacts to being interviewed. Some parents have been quite skilled in assessing what part of public life their child is seeking as well as creative in addressing this need.

After talking to several public children in our clinic, Mark, a young boy, repeatedly asked that he be able to "give lectures and do TV shows." His mother was reluctant to pursue public appearances because Mark was developmentally delayed, had occasional behavioral problems, and had difficulties adjusting to changes in routine. When Mark was asked why he wanted to be on TV, he replied, "Because I want to ride in a limousine." Mark's mother responded by hiring a limousine for a few hours one afternoon.

The child's disease severity may be another factor affecting the decision to go public. An important question is whether the child has the physical and emotional reserves to adequately deal with publicity. As the child's disease progresses, physical, emotional, and intellectual fatigue is often present. Powell-Cope and Brown (1992) reviewed considerations that family caregivers have given for going public and found that the most significant influence on the timing and staging of such disclosure was the health status of the person with AIDS. This was not discussed by the children or their parents in the present study, and it is an important issue to consider. Does the child feel that his or her time is limited and feel the need to "make a difference"? Such discussions could help the child feel less alone with his or her thoughts, fears, and/or anxieties associated with progressive disease. The decision to go public can then be understood as the need to leave something of oneself behind or to make a difference while one still can. Powell-Cope and Brown also found that caregivers' activism in AIDS was motivated by a desire to create social change, to demonstrate self-pride, and to affirm a belief that they could make a difference in society's response to HIV. This was clearly described by the children and their parents.

For those families who do choose to be open with their diagnosis in the mass media, we recommend that the clinician help them explore possible negative consequences prior to the disclosure, as well as exploring effective means of dealing with such outcomes. Many families have reported situations to us in which they felt that their story was presented inaccurately or were displeased by the angle taken by the media. Examples include a focus on the eventual death of the child, portraying the child as a "victim," and portraying the child as being more healthy and as having fewer problems than was the case. To some extent, all families in the public eye—to varying degrees—lose control over what is presented and the slant of the presentation. Almost 50% of our parental sample reported that on at least one occasion, they had felt "used" by a member of the mass media. All of the children reported at least one experience where they felt a sense of rejection after spending hours with a reporter only to be given a few seconds on television. Helping to prepare a child for this eventuality is of critical importance.

Having a public child in the family can arouse many different feelings in other siblings, especially HIV-negative siblings in the household. Although parents and children did not report worsening of relationships within the family following public disclosure, it is not uncommon for these siblings to describe feelings of being ignored and unimportant. This is not a trivial issue, as healthy siblings of chronically ill children tend to report such feelings regularly, and the feelings are likely to be intensified by public attention for the ill child. For example, the well child must

compete for attention with a "famous" sibling, which could either moti-
vate the well sibling to high achievement or lay the groundwork for disturbances of the self (Fanos & Wiener, 1994).

Occasionally, public families suffer from negative and sometimes
hostile responses from others. We have had patients whose public disclosure resulted in their being banned from school or church or their home
being vandalized or targeted for hate mail, among other things. Unfortunately, these outcomes must be considered. Finally, the parents must
be alerted to look for any signs or symptoms in their child that would
suggest that public exposure should be discontinued or decreased. We
had one child develop facial tics after doing several lectures, news interviews, and other TV exposures. Specifically, parents should look for
changes in appetite or sleep patterns not related to the HIV, changes in
mood, self-destructive or acting-out behavior, or withdrawal from previously enjoyable activities, along with any of the common symptoms of
anxiety or depression.

▓ Conclusions

Despite the stigma that has clouded HIV/AIDS since it was first identified in the United States in 1981, most families struggle to find ways to
communicate the diagnosis to their children. Disclosure styles vary
greatly and range from those who choose not to share the diagnosis with
siblings or with extended family members, let alone friends and neighbors, to those who share the child's diagnosis with the community. In
recent years, a limited number of families have decided to bring their
family plight to the attention of the media. This chapter highlights the
emotional turmoil these public families faced in deciding whether or not
to go public and the sequelae associated with living a public life. Most
have reported their experience to be a positive one and, if provided the
opportunity, would go public all over again. Clearly, many other families
will follow in their footsteps.

The findings in the present study suggest that public children perceive themselves as having a lower sense of social, scholastic, physical,
and global self-competence than children who have not disclosed their
diagnosis to the media. There is a trend for these families to report fewer
social supports and more family conflict. However, the stress of the com-

bination of living with a life-threatening disease, losing one's parents and friends to the same disease, and knowing that so many "eyes" are watching how one responds to these events should not be underestimated. These children are often raised to the status of hero, and stories such as "Child Dying With AIDS Gives Inspirational Talk to College Students" may be particularly difficult to endure at a time when the child's internal experience may be so discrepant (Libow, 1992).

Despite the potential undesirable effects, there were many beneficial experiences that the children and families related to us about being public. They enjoyed the freedom afforded to them in terms of being open about the disease. They have often received tremendous praise for their courage. Letters and calls offering hope, social support, and for some, financial assistance have been invaluable. Many of these children received unsolicited gifts, offers to meet famous entertainers, and trips to places they never would have visited if not for their publicity. Most of all, they report being proud of how they have been able to help others and of the fact that they have joined the forces of people fighting this disease. The accolades, praise, and confirmation associated with public disclosure become part of their emotional identity as the disease defines their physical state. It is the responsibility of the child's parent(s) or guardian(s) as well as the health care team to help balance the families' motivations and altruistic desires with the practical and psychosocial ramifications associated with living a public life.

▓ Notes

1. Refers to the outpatient clinic at the Pediatric Branch of the National Cancer Institute, where children participate in HIV-related clinical trials. Each child and family are also offered mental health services as part of their care.

2. Public families scored an average of 10.3 ($SD = 5.19$) on the BDI and nonpublic families scored 10.2 ($SD = .77$). According to Beck and Steer (1987), scores of 0 to 9 represent individuals who are asymptomatic for depression, scores of 10 to 18 indicate mild to moderate depression, scores of 19 to 29 indicate moderate to severe depression, and scores of 30 to 63 indicate extremely severe depression. Within normal populations, scores of greater than 15 are thought to detect possible depression.

An Eye to the Future of HIV/AIDS and Social Relationships
An Epilogue

KATHRYN GREENE
East Carolina University, Greenville

JULIANNE M. SEROVICH
Ohio State University, Columbus

The social consequences of the HIV/AIDS epidemic have gone unrecognized for too long. Researchers of HIV/AIDS have for years examined drug regimens, treatments, and transmission of HIV, but far less work has examined the relationships of people with HIV/AIDS and how people with HIV/AIDS live with the disease. Our hope is that the chapters in this book help to fill this gap by presenting a range of research regarding social interaction and HIV/AIDS. This book has addressed how an HIV-positive person interacts with others and the effect of HIV on how others respond to an HIV-positive person.

With new treatments, people with HIV/AIDS are living longer, even further reinforcing the need to study social aspects of HIV/AIDS. It may be that, with increased awareness, more people are also aware of diagnoses earlier in the course of the disease and are receiving health care earlier (HIV testing has increased, even giving rise to a new home-based test). Very little research is presently available that explores the relationships of those who are HIV positive. Much investigation of health problems has occurred previously, but less attention has been given to increasing the psychological, emotional, and relational quality of the lives of people with HIV/AIDS.

Effect of New Treatments

At the XI International Conference on AIDS (Vancouver, Canada, 1996), physicians and researchers from around the world began to speak about a possible eradication of the deadly disease. Scientists met to discuss new treatment strategies and medical regimens for HIV-positive persons. This created, for the first time in 15 years, cautious optimism in a community battling a disease that has debilitated and killed millions around the world. This unprecedented optimism has come from the work of researchers experimenting with new drug combinations often referred to as antiretroviral therapies, more commonly known as cocktail therapies (which include protease inhibitors). The most beneficial aspect of this treatment is that, for some patients, viral load (the amount of virus in the body) can be reduced to extraordinarily low levels or become virtually undetectable in the bloodstream. Many HIV-positive individuals have experienced a rebound in immune functioning with these therapies. If the virus can be caught early enough and the individual is receptive to treatment, HIV-positive people may be expected to live much longer, experience fewer associated illnesses, and maintain a higher quality of life.

These new therapies do, however, have associated difficulties (see Greene & Cassidy, in press). First, the availability of treatment is limited and very expensive. Typically, at present, only those individuals employed by private companies, enrolled in federally funded clinical trials, or with access to subsidies for medications receive treatment. Second, some researchers have found antiretroviral treatment does not work for certain strains of the disease. Third, because of the toxicity of the drug combinations, side effects for some persons are near intolerable levels (e.g., nausea). Finally, being treated with antiretroviral therapies requires individuals to adhere to very strict and sometimes cumbersome treatment protocols. Because noncompliance can quickly result in the virus becoming drug resistant, patients are forced to carefully monitor and maintain demanding dosage schedules. Despite the drawbacks of the new antiretroviral drug therapies, it is possible with these medical advances that HIV/AIDS may become a chronic condition rather than a fatal illness. At first glance, then, the news appears to be very positive: HIV-positive people may live longer, fuller, and healthier lives. If it is true that HIV/AIDS will become a chronic, manageable disease, what issues will infected persons confront?

A number of the social issues facing HIV-positive persons have been addressed in this book. For example, disclosure of an HIV-positive diagnosis continues to be an important issue for HIV-positive persons. If HIV/AIDS becomes chronic, disclosure may become even more consequential. How will helping professionals persuade HIV-positive persons to disclose to a sexual partner when the threat of imminent death is no longer attached to the disease? If rates of disclosure to family members and friends decrease, how will the infected person be able to access social support? If the stigma associated with HIV/AIDS is dependent on perceived control of infection, then stigma is unlikely to change for quite some time.

This epilogue will first discuss research in the book by summarizing findings presented for stigma, self disclosure, coping, social support, and identity; the social interaction model of coping with HIV infection presented by Derlega and Barbee (Chapter 1) provides a way to understand how these variables are interrelated. Next, we will cover implications for groups such as therapists, health care practitioners, community organizations, message designers, and policy makers. Finally, we will look at conclusions and directions for future research on social consequences of HIV infection.

■ Summary of Social Interaction Themes for HIV-Infected Persons

Taking the chapters together, there were five main themes that emerged as important social issues surrounding HIV/AIDS. People who are HIV infected struggle with stigma, self-disclosure, coping, social support, and identity issues, and these are crucial in their relationships and in the model of coping with HIV infection developed by Derlega and Barbee (Chapter 1). This section focuses only on social or relational variables and includes other factors (e.g., depression) only in relation to their effect on social relationships. The variables discussed include stigma, self-disclosure, coping, social support, and identity.

Stigma

AIDS has been labeled the most controversial disease in modern history (Powell-Cope & Brown, 1992), and HIV-infected persons report that facing stigma is one of their greatest challenges and sources of stress (see Chapter 2). Reactions to HIV-infected persons are influenced by who is infected as well as how they are infected. There is a misperception that HIV/AIDS can only be contracted through stigmatized behaviors (see Chapter 1), initially male-to-male sex and intravenous drug use. There has also been slippage where the categories of gay, promiscuous, and AIDS have collapsed or become nearly synonymous (see McAllister, 1992; Watney, 1987). The news coverage of AIDS has clearly contributed to this stigma. As Watney (1986) noted, "A disease of chimpanzees or gerbils would have attracted more sympathetic coverage" (p. 47). HIV-infected persons must deal not only with the disease and their feelings but the reactions of others.

Deviance is often labeled as illness, and certain illnesses carry meanings other than biomedical, such that the illness becomes a metaphor for characteristics attributed to the person (McAllister, 1992; Sontag, 1979). One central component separating HIV/AIDS stigma (except, for example, leprosy) is potential threat to the health of another. Fear of contagion (sometimes based on lack of knowledge about transmission) remains despite extensive public awareness campaigns. The public association of AIDS with risk *groups* rather than risk *behaviors* remains, as has been the case since early in the epidemic.

Stigma includes a group focus in which the differences of a group are emphasized rather than its similarities to other groups. This tendency to emphasize the differences between groups and similarities within groups (especially in the outgroup) is known as the outgroup homogeneity effect (see Mullen & Hu, 1989; Ostrom & Sedikides, 1992). Understanding this process is crucial in explaining stereotyping and stigma: "Some cultural groups sustain themselves by assigning positive traits and rewards to their group (ingroup), while assigning unfavorable traits and potential punishments to outside groups" (Michal-Johnson &

Bowen, 1992, p. 161). People typically judge the group to which they belong (the ingroup) as being more variable and positive than the group to which they do not belong (the outgroup). The result of this outgroup homogeneity bias is that members of the outgroup are all perceived as being alike. This lack of perceived group variability leads to stereotyping, and this is a good way to understand how the concepts "gay man" and "HIV positive" have become equated.

AIDS stigma has also led to labeling and blame, focusing on responsibility for the disease (see Chapter 2). Attributions about stigma are often based on perception of control over infection. Stigma seen as uncontrollable evokes more favorable responses, but stigma perceived as controllable evokes very negative responses. This kind of control stigma can be seen in popular terminology labeling children as "innocent victims," and this has created a victim continuum (innocent versus deserving) in some perceptions. It may be that stigma is a way to disassociate or create distance for some through assignment of responsibility to those infected. If people do not participate in the blaming behaviors, they may be able to convince themselves they are not at risk.

Another interesting concept not well explored in the literature but addressed in this book is "courtesy stigma." People who are closely associated with HIV-infected persons also get stigmatized, mostly in negative ways (see Chapter 2). In Chapter 6, this is identified as stigma by association, affecting volunteers who work with HIV-infected persons. This can hold true not just for family members and friends but also for health care providers and workers, social workers, and therapists who treat or work with HIV-infected persons. HIV-serodiscordant couples are yet another example of those dealing with the association effects of stigma (Chapter 9). Merely associating with HIV-infected persons can bring about the same kinds of stigma that targets HIV-infected persons. Courtesy stigma may be the basis for some people avoiding HIV-infected persons (fear association), possibly leading to distance from friends, family, and others. This courtesy association is not unique to AIDS (though it is probably more intense); for example, families with incarcerated members or an alcoholic member often go to great lengths to conceal these facts.

HIV/AIDS-related stigma runs through many chapters in this book, and stigma is central to Derlega and Barbee's (Chapter 1) model of coping with HIV infection. Perhaps one of most insidious effects of AIDS-related stigma, apart from lack of opportunity to gain social support for those infected, has been hesitancy to disclose. Failure to disclose sero-status is one of the causes of the continuation of the epidemic because it means failure to notify others (e.g., sexual or needle-sharing partners) of their risk for infection and, simultaneously, self-denial of opportunity to gain social support. Next, we will turn to how HIV-positive people deal with issues of disclosure.

Self-Disclosure

The initial response of many is to keep an HIV-positive diagnosis a secret. One of the consequences of AIDS-related stigma can be nondisclosure and potentially decreased social support, with possible negative physical and psychological health effects (Chapter 2). Kimberly, Serovich, and Greene (1995) reported that HIV-positive women experienced an initial stage in the disclosure process of telling no one, often corresponding to several months of nondisclosure. There is a growing body of research on how people decide who to tell about their HIV infection (see Chapter 8; Greene & Serovich, 1996; Hays et al., 1992; Marks, Bundek, et al., 1992; Serovich, Kimberly, & Greene, 1998). Findings indicate that people disclose their HIV/AIDS status very selectively.

There are benefits and risks to self-disclosure, and people must balance the competing need to maintain privacy and control and the need to share information (Chapter 8). HIV-positive individuals struggle with decisions to disclose in such a way that they may receive support but avoid negative consequences associated with AIDS (see Greene & Serovich, 1996; Yep, 1993). Clearly, disclosure is a double-edged sword: It is possible to lose social support through disclosure, yet potential support can also be eliminated through failure to disclose (Hays et al., 1992). Benefits from disclosing include such things as feeling loved and accepted, gaining information, and making safer sex decisions. Conversely, there are risks for HIV-positive individuals who disclose their serostatus, and decisions to disclose are likely to be filled with fear and anxiety (Marks, Bundek, et al., 1992; Yep, 1993). The potential impact of such disclosures is wide ranging, from ostracism in interpersonal relationships to self-identity crises, from threats to basic survival (loss of employment, housing, insurance, or health care) to loss of social support. People must see benefits in disclosure before being willing to expose themselves (Hays et al., 1992).

Petronio's (1991) theory of boundary management (similar to the analysis of privacy regulation in Chapter 8) describes how people control potential risk to self when disclosing. Individuals erect a metaphoric boundary to protect themselves and reduce their chances of losing face. The risks associated with disclosing HIV infection are tremendous, perhaps leading to more rigid boundaries (little or no disclosure). Yep (1993) applied this theory specifically to the potential vulnerability of disclosure of HIV infection. Because disclosure is a relational event, variables associated with both the sender and receiver need to be examined (Yep, 1993). Data presented in this book (Chapters 8 and 10) show how individuals must perceive a positive response or some benefit from disclosure before they are willing to disclose.

Although we know more about disclosure of HIV infection than previously, little is known about *how* disclosure choices are made. It is likely that these decisions are made after careful consideration and with a great deal of selectivity (see Greene & Serovich, 1996; Marks, Bundek, et al., 1992; Simoni et al., 1995; Yep, 1993). The factors in decisions to disclose to one target person (e.g., mother) are likely to be different than those used in deciding on another (e.g., partner). Members of the marital subsystem (lovers, spouses, ex-spouses, friends) have been viewed as the most appropriate targets for disclosure of HIV infection, with the nuclear family (e.g., parents, siblings, children) rating next highest (Greene & Serovich, 1996; Marks, Bundek, et al., 1992; Serovich & Greene, 1993; Simoni et al., 1995); lowest-rated targets were extended family and the general public.

Serovich, Greene, and Parrott (1992) looked at the potential recipient of HIV-testing information. Individuals overall reported most desire to restrict access to HIV-testing information to the general public, less to the community, and least (or more access) to the marital subsystem. Serovich and Greene (1993) expanded this work by looking at potential family targets for release of HIV-testing information. Overall, participants reported most support for access to HIV-testing information to the marital system (e.g., lovers, spouses), moderate to the nuclear family (e.g., mother, son), and least to the extended family (e.g., aunt, mother-in-law). Greene and Serovich (1996) replicated these studies and reported HIV-infected persons also have clear distinctions in perceptions of appropriate recipients of information about HIV infection. In addition, HIV-infected persons reported less desire (compared with other groups) for disclosure of HIV infection across all subsystems. Similarly,

Marks, Bundek, et al. (1992) reported that HIV-positive persons were highly selective in choosing targets of disclosure and tended to inform significant others (parents, friends, and lovers) more than nonsignificant others (employers, landlords, and religious leaders).

Expectations regarding partner's response is the first factor a discloser takes into account before sharing (Petronio, 1991). Kimberly et al. (1995) reported that women specifically cited the expected response from the target as a reason for disclosing or not disclosing their HIV infection. If a person anticipates that the recipient will respond negatively (e.g., with hostility, judgmentally, or with ignorance) or neutrally to disclosure, she or he will probably choose to withhold the information. It may be necessary, given a topic as sensitive as AIDS, for a person to be relatively certain of a positive response before disclosing HIV infection.

Perception of a relationship is also likely to be a significant determinant of willingness to disclose HIV infection. In addition to the role a relationship (for example, sister) plays, the quality of that relationship is likely to differentiate relationships. For example, a person can have varying degrees of relational qualities with a sister, and this perception of the relationship may be a deciding factor in disclosure. A person would be unlikely to disclose information as sensitive as HIV infection to someone with whom she or he had a poor relationship.

Disclosure may be a means of obtaining social support, and social support may serve a significant role in mediating between stress and health (Albrecht & Adelman, 1987c; Greenblatt, Becerra, & Serafetinides, 1982). Disclosure of traumatic experiences has been reported to reduce stress (Greenberg & Stone, 1992; Pennebaker, 1989) and physical and mental health problems (Pennebaker, 1990; Susman, 1988). In addition, satisfaction with social support among HIV-positive men increases both psychological (Kelly, Chu, & Buehler, 1993; Zich & Temoshok, 1987) and physical (Hays et al., 1992; Zich & Temoshok, 1987) well-being.

This book has provided significant information that will contribute to understanding how disclosure functions for HIV-positive people. Disclosure may play a helpful role in coping with disease and diagnosis by opening opportunities for support but may add stress due to stigmatization, discrimination, and relationship disruption (see Chapter 8). Next, we will discuss research presented on coping with HIV.

Coping

Coping with HIV/AIDS is important in understanding social interactions for HIV-infected people. Problem-solving coping is generally associated with positive health and medical conditions; avoidant coping is
generally associated with psychological distress and poor outcomes (see
Chapter 9). Avoidant coping may have some positive short-term effects,
but long-term adjustment is associated with approach-oriented coping
(see results of the meta-analysis by Suls & Fletcher, 1985).

There are contradictions in the literature on the effects of illness on
relationships. Clearly factors of stress and resources are crucial in determining the effects of HIV on relationships. Disrupted relationships have
been documented as responses to the burden of HIV infection (Chapter
9). HIV/AIDS affects not only the infected person but those close to him
or her, especially partners, family, and friends. There is not as much
research on the effects of HIV/AIDS for partners of infected persons (for
exceptions, see Chapter 9 and Folkman, 1997), although relational quality is thought to be one of the most important components in coping with
relationships.

Relationships are affected differently by illness at different stages.
Coping is expected to vary with stage of disease for both the partner and
the infected person. The initial effects of HIV infection may include less
physical disturbance but more psychological stress; later, physical and
financial stress may increase as well. Moore et al. (Chapter 9) found that
increased disease stage leads to more depressive symptoms such that
both members of a couple are negatively affected by the illness.

This book points to the need for more study on progression or stages
of coping (Chapter 1). It would be expected that, with changes in disease
progression, coping might need to shift. With newer treatments, these
coping strategies may become even more important. Next, we will discuss research presented on social support.

Social Support

Potential sources of support for HIV-infected people can be lost
through nondisclosure, stigma, or negative coping strategies. There are
different kinds of social support, often dichotomized as instrumental
(e.g., money or child care) and expressive (e.g., affection or sympathy).

Physical and mental effects of social support have been documented, with less social support related to more depression and increased social support linked with better health. The unmet social support needs for HIV-infected persons, along with the collapse of traditional institutions that are supposed to provide support (see Dane & Miller, 1992), have created a need for innovative kinds of structures and groups to provide services (see Chapter 7).

Distressed people have a general idea of the form of support they want (see sensitive interaction systems theory, Chapter 5), but these support needs are not always met. A common response to HIV infection is lack of social support from family members (see Metts, Manns, & Kruzic, 1996). HIV-infected persons often feel abandoned by families, and in gay communities, social networks have been ravaged by AIDS. In response to absence of support, AIDS organizations began to provide self-help groups. As of this writing, there is limited documentation of the effectiveness of such groups, although they provide both formal and informal support (see Chapter 7).

HIV-infected persons receive support from a range of people. Friends' and health care workers' support is generally perceived as helpful, but lovers were viewed as mixed on helpfulness. Interestingly, not much family support was viewed as helpful. Barbee et al. (Chapter 5) provide details about what constituted unhelpful support, such as escape behaviors and dismiss or avoidant behaviors, and unhelpful solace. Specific recommendations for helpful behaviors are also provided. These findings indicate that well-meaning people (especially family) can botch attempts at support; Barbee et al. recommend asking HIV-infected persons what kind of support would be helpful.

One of the strengths of this book in terms of social support may be the specific identification of failed attempts at social support. This can provide guidelines for those attempting to offer support. Partners and family members generally want to be supportive; however, social support interactions can sometimes be less than helpful. Family members dealing with their own sense of impending loss and grief may not be in the best place to offer the support desired by HIV-infected persons. Social support in the form of advice, tangible assistance, and emotional support will not always be wanted or helpful (Chapter 5). Social support will remain a crucial issue for HIV-infected persons. Next, we will discuss research presented on identity.

Identity

Based on what was been reviewed earlier (stigma, self-disclosure di-lemmas, coping problems, and loss of social support), it appears that HIV-infected persons need social support to restore or bolster self-es-teem, create meaning during crisis, and gain control over their lives. Formal support can have a positive effect on identity, and formal support groups can increase a positive sense of self (Chapter 7).

For HIV-infected persons, one goal is normal treatment (Chapter 2). Stigmatized people have lower self-esteem, and stigma may be a stressor that leads HIV-infected persons to commit suicide. Identity is central for HIV-infected persons, and they often end up "passing" and covering to protect their identity. Being stigmatized may also function to protect one's self-esteem (Crocker & Major, 1989) because any negative feed-back can be attributed to their HIV infection (Chapter 10). The effect of others' reactions on self-esteem and self-concept cannot be underesti-mated.

In this section, we have discussed research presented in the book for stigma, self-disclosure, coping, social support, and identity. Each of these variables is discussed in different chapters and plays a significant role in social aspects of HIV and in the model presented by Derlega and Barbee (Chapter 1). All of this research leads to a better understanding of the social consequences of HIV infection.

Special Issues for HIV-Positive Persons, Their Families, and Helping Professionals

In this section, we will discuss how the information presented in this book can help HIV-positive persons and their significant others in coping with HIV/AIDS. In addition, the information presented may help profes-sionals such as therapists and health care workers assist HIV-positive persons and their family and friends. The information can also be used by HIV/AIDS community organizations, HIV message designers, and public policy makers.

As a reminder, each subpopulation infected with HIV is different and cannot always be discussed together because perspectives of the dis-ease and needs are different by group (see Chapter 3). For example, in Chapter 4, Rose indicates that black gay men create meanings of HIV that may be different from others; therefore, the process by which they cope with their infection and are affected by stigma is very different from that of white gay men. Similarly, Hispanic females experienced higher levels of depression and less intimacy in their relationships compared with white or black women (see Chapter 9). Therefore, it is imperative that implications and suggestions made here are used only in light of the person in individual context.

HIV-Positive Persons

As we mentioned in the beginning of this chapter, for people living with HIV/AIDS, this is an optimistic, exciting, yet challenging time. New medical therapies and treatment possibilities are proliferating at a rapid pace. Although hope prevails, the somber reality is that a cure has not yet been developed. Until a cure is available and HIV is eradicated, there are a number of recommendations that emerged from the research in this book that might be particularly helpful for HIV-positive persons as they cope with their illness. HIV/AIDS is more than a medical phenomenon, as it has significant social implications.

Obtaining social support is imperative for both the emotional and physical health of HIV-infected people. Support can be garnered from professionals, personal social contacts, or through community agencies. Professional support can be in the form of psychotherapy, spiritual guidance, or other healing specialists. HIV-positive individuals may experience support from friends, formal or informal support groups, and/or community organizations as being the most beneficial. Extending the social support network beyond partners and family members will be crucial. This is especially important if HIV takes on a more chronic, long-term nature because the role of support groups and other formal systems of support may need to be used to an even greater degree.

Along with social support, the coping strategies HIV-positive persons adopt play significant roles in psychological adaptation. More specifically, active coping strategies appear to be more helpful than avoidant coping strategies. Active coping strategies include developing problem-solving abilities and help-seeking behaviors as well as acquiring information-seeking and verification skills. Each of these approaches indirectly promotes self-reliance, self-respect, and the development of optimism. Although avoidant coping behaviors might produce short-term relief, HIV-positive persons are encouraged to seek programs that offer problem-solving-focused skill development. Likewise, helping professionals should offer programs with an active-coping-based curriculum to help HIV-positive persons better handle stressful situations.

One way active coping skills can be used is with medical personnel. Because changing medical protocols can be confusing and cumbersome, HIV-positive persons need to develop strategies for obtaining clear and concise medical information from health professionals. This includes information about available treatment options and the consequences associated with each protocol as well as any associated side effects. For example, many treatment protocols have medication schedules that are quite complex and confusing. New routines around meals and sleep may clash with established work or leisure schedules. Because compliance with medication schedules is required for satisfactory medical results, the ability to gather this information is imperative for HIV-positive persons. Thus, active coping skills may be pivotal for persons to feel in control of their medical treatment and demand the most accurate information.

Family Members and Significant Others

Throughout the book a few general conclusions emerged concerning family members of HIV-positive individuals. Family members are not always viewed as particularly helpful to HIV-positive persons. Before drawing conclusions about family members too quickly, however, several issues should be addressed. As Leary and Schreindorfer (Chapter 2) point out, HIV-positive persons experience direct results of stigma, but family members can be stigmatized by association. Therefore, for some family members, the externalized result of stigma by association might be the appearance of being cold and unfeeling. If this is the case, family members might find solace in support group or therapy settings.

Furthermore, if we accept Rose's conclusion in Chapter 4 that helping HIV-positive persons derive meaning from their association with HIV is useful, then a similar strategy might be used for family members. Family members might search to derive meaning from having an HIV-infected member and by doing so help to acknowledge the fear, sorrow, and anger they might harbor. It is also possible that family members lack the knowledge and skills to assist the HIV-positive member. If this is the case, family intervention strategies might include the provision of support groups, which could serve as a source of information about HIV, support for personal grieving, and the opportunity to develop effective helping skills. Family members must seek social support themselves, not just for the infected person, especially if they are primary caregivers.

Both partners and HIV-infected individuals become more depressed as the disease progresses (Chapter 9). Given this, significant others must not ignore their own mental health and coping difficulties. In fact, both members of a couple, despite the HIV status of either individual, should seek clinical assessments, interventions, and follow-ups routinely. Efforts made to provide support groups for partners and spouses should be encouraged and tailored to different couple types. For example, support groups for gay male partners would involve significantly different issues from those for interracial, heterosexual, or lesbian couples.

Many children of HIV-infected women may be hidden victims of this disease. Some mothers may be unable to accurately assess the needs of their children due to being overwhelmed, overburdened, and/or depressed. Others, mainly therapists and health care workers, will have to be aware of the needs of these children and make sure the children are adequately cared for both emotionally and physically. Overall, the results of these studies bring to light the need for therapists to take a global and systemic view of the life of HIV-positive persons to make sure the overall health of their families and networks are being served. If the needs of these networks are met and satisfied, it is plausible that the mental and physical health of HIV-positive persons will also be positively affected.

Helping Professionals

Helping professionals is defined here as any professionally trained mental health worker, including individual counselors, social workers, psychotherapists, psychiatrists, and marriage and family therapists. Helping professionals may also be health care practitioners and HIV/AIDS service organization workers. Furthermore, *client* can mean not only an HIV-positive person but a partner or spouse, family member, or friend.

The work presented in this book gives therapists guidance for developing more sophisticated skills and treatment plans for working with HIV-positive persons and their support networks. For example, Collins (Chapter 3) points out that support received from the gay community is very important for various coping outcomes for HIV-infected gay men.

She found gay pride positively related to having a constructive life focus and the development of new relationships. Furthermore, having pride in being homosexual was strongly associated with several indicators of coping and social support. Therefore, therapists should assess the degree to which gay men are connected with the gay community and assist with social identification whenever possible. Undoubtedly, encouraging HIV-positive men who are homosexual to reach out and become involved in the gay community may be a treatment strategy that is underused. Helping professionals should be aware, however, that because of stigma there may be a tendency for some to withdraw from the gay community. Helping professionals should help clients resist withdrawing from community interaction and support.

Derlega et al. (Chapter 8) provide therapists and health care workers with useful tips and guidelines when working with HIV-positive persons around the process of disclosure. The reasons for disclosure provided by Derlega et al. can help therapists explore with clients reasons, fears, expectations, successes, and doubts about disclosing. For example, therapists working with newly diagnosed individuals as they struggle with competing disclosure needs could empower clients with reasons why others have chosen to disclose or not disclose. Therapists could also facilitate discussion of effective steps in the disclosure process (see Kimberly et al., 1995) and reactions of family members to disclosure of an HIV-positive diagnosis (Serovich et al., 1998). In fact, provision of each of these experiences of others can help HIV-positive clients further clarify their own decision-making processes.

Health care workers are frequently the bearers of bad news to HIV-positive persons. Typically, initial diagnoses, test results, and difficult treatment decisions are shared by and with doctors, nurses, and/or social workers. Because the implications of many of these decisions are difficult and painful, health care practitioners can find themselves offering solace to grieving patients and family members. Professionals should attempt to provide very practical assistance, such as suggestions for how to solve a particular problem, or be emotionally available and reassuring of patients (Chapter 5).

If new treatment regimens are as beneficial for a longer life as promised, then health care workers and helping professionals will be building longer relationships with their patients. In fact, health care workers are likely to become emotionally closer and more involved with patients by helping them comply with medication schedules and assisting with strategies for handling complicated side effects. Health care workers are also more likely to become sources of information and referral on related matters such as nutrition and exercise. Health care workers will need to be more equipped with helpful strategies to assist patients. In addition, hospital social workers or therapists should be aware of the emotional needs of health care workers as they become more entwined with the lives of patients.

Public Education Campaigns

Public education campaign designers can play a key role in the fight against stigma surrounding intravenous drug users, sex workers, homosexuals, and others considered "marked." Stigma management strategies for public education campaigns can be successful if they reduce notions that HIV-positive persons "pose a threat" to the health and well-being of others, deviate from group standards, do not contribute to society, or elicit negative emotions (Chapter 2). An example of an HIV-positive person being portrayed in positive light is a Nike running shoe advertisement that features an HIV-positive marathon runner. In this advertisement the runner is obviously health conscious, appears to enjoy a particular sport, and is ambitious. Here is a positive portrayal of an HIV-infected person following a dream undeterred by his infection. Messages in the form of advertisements, health promotion campaigns, or public education messages that emphasize positive qualities of HIV-infected persons should be encouraged and supported.

The relationship between stigma and homophobia arises in many of these chapters. Therefore, campaigns to reduce the fear of homosexuals should be pervasive and should target populations shown to be more homophobic than others. For example, as Rose (Chapter 4) points out, homophobia may be especially prevalent in minority, ethnic, or underserved populations. Men are also more likely than women to express negative attitudes toward homosexual men (Kite & Whitley, 1996). Given these findings, public education campaigns should be directed toward outlets such as churches, magazines, or other venues with a large ethnic or male following. In effect, specifically targeted anti-homophobia campaigns are needed to help reduce AIDS-related stigma.

It is also important to remember that besides reducing stigma in the general public, positive messages can help families and HIV-positive persons in reducing stigma. If stigma damages many more people than those infected, as Leary and Schreindorfer (Chapter 2) suggest, campaigns may be the most important tool for fighting stigma. Because it is unlikely that new treatment regimes will significantly reduce the stigma associated with homosexuality and HIV, public education about sexual orientation issues is important.

Community HIV/AIDS Organizations

Community HIV/AIDS organizations are the front-line source of support, education, resources, and information for HIV-positive persons, family, and friends, as well as the general public. Obviously, their work would be costly and burdensome without the help of volunteers who fill the roles of buddies, community speakers, and risk-reduction specialists. For many organizations, these persons are the backbone of the organization and unquestionably the driving force behind the fight against the spread of HIV.

There are a number of implications from this book that are applicable specifically to community organizations. Helpers/volunteers should be adequately prepared for the fact that relationship quality between helper and client diminishes over time (Chapter 6). Training for volunteers, no matter their role, should incorporate a sense of realism about what to expect, including personality clashes, lack of client appreciation, and possible client death. Preparation could be accomplished by having experienced buddies and HIV-positive persons speak directly to this issue at training group meetings.

HIV-prevention programming clearly needs to be tailored to specific communities of people. A strategy or program designed for gay men might not work or have relevant characteristics for black gay men, older adolescents, or women. Although a contextual approach to prevention efforts is important, certain successful characteristics of HIV programming with one population are worth experimenting with in others. For example, according to Rose (Chapter 4), programs that increase self-esteem, self-worth, and provide meaning for gay men tend to increase optimism and self-respect. Although increasing self-esteem in gay men was found to be important, such results could also have a significant impact for women, children, or African American male populations. The mechanism by which such components are incorporated into programming efforts need to be contextually sensitive and deserves further research attention.

Much like health care workers, if HIV/AIDS becomes a chronic illness, community organizational staff are likely to become more involved in the lives of HIV-positive clients. In addition, new interventions and strategies for helping their clients deal with disease uncertainty, obtaining new drug therapies, disclosure, and stigma will have to be developed and implemented.

Public Policy and HIV Prevention

There are implications for health message design from these chapters. Stigma associated with HIV/AIDS may contribute to unwillingness to disclose HIV infection or reduced social support. More effort to reduce stereotypes will be crucial in controlling the spread of HIV/AIDS. The moral problems associated with HIV/AIDS are complicated by the effects of social stigma and labeling. Specific campaigns portraying how families are affected by HIV/AIDS and the support families can provide might be useful in reducing this stigma and labeling. There is also evidence that different messages should be created for women and men and, probably, messages that differ by race and sexual orientation as well.

Reducing stigma is quite a challenge, as it will require undoing decades of policy (e.g., as it has with race relations). One example of a stigma-reduction intervention was quite successful. Monteith (1993) gave feedback to undergraduates about their prejudice, making their homophobia seem nonnormative, and was able to demonstrate later reduction in prejudiced attitudes. It might be possible to use the same sort of technique with HIV-positive persons. To reduce stigma, forcing people to confront disassociation views might also work: for example, requiring people to interact with HIV-infected persons.

Conclusions and Future Research

Providing conclusions for a book on the social aspects of HIV is a difficult task, as HIV/AIDS continues to change. New information about treatments may cause significant shifts in many relationships described here, as this is a rapidly changing area. Even with new and radically different treatments, however, the contributions of these chapters are especially significant because they focus on how people with HIV interact with others and how others respond in light of their HIV infection. One aspect consistent in this work was the role of stigma and how stigma could vary by subgroup. Stigma affects how HIV-infected people live with the disease, specifically their disclosure, social support, coping strategies, and identity.

There is a need to continue to examine the role of gender in social aspects of HIV/AIDS. Women and men are clearly affected by HIV/AIDS differently, from coping strategies to media images. Over 50% of HIV-positive women have children under the age of 18 (Ickovics & Rodin, 1992), and this will be crucial to consider. Yet, there has been only limited systematic research on women (for exceptions, see books since 1994). The gay community is also discussed rather thoroughly in this book, but there is no mention of the effect of HIV/AIDS on lesbians. Lesbians form significant portions of volunteer networks, and the "gay community" label may overlook their role. The Fall 1996 issue of *Women's Health* was devoted to lesbians and HIV/AIDS, but even so, more than black gay men, heterosexual women, or children, lesbians with HIV/AIDS are invisible.

Demographic findings related to HIV/AIDS can also be overlooked in attempts to see patterns or similarities in HIV-infected persons. Researchers must look at junctures including such issues as income, race, and gender. For example, who pays for medications, and with what insurance? New treatment options provide great promise, but is it possible that new treatments will be used primarily with certain racial or socio-economic groups? All of these questions point to the continued importance of considering demographics. Race differences are important because they have created invisible groups of HIV-infected persons. An example highlighted in this book is black gay men who face unique challenges in confronting their infection. It is easy to downplay the role of economic factors and lack of formal education, but not often mentioned are sexual abuse, physical abuse, and drug or alcohol addiction (see Chapter 4).

Cultural differences are also not well understood in HIV infection generally. As Michal-Johnson and Bowen (1992) state, "HIV has had a far more profound effect in communities of color and in the gay community than in any others in the United States" (p. 147). If culture is to be an organizing concept for AIDS interventions, clearly AIDS public service announcements do not meet this standard (see Freimuth, Hammond, Edgar, & Monahan, 1990). Freimuth et al.'s content analysis of AIDS public service announcements shows that they are targeted for general audiences and avoid explicit language, and this clearly does not meet long-standing recommendations for culturally sensitive, group-specific prevention messages.

With new treatments for HIV/AIDS changing rapidly, it seems imperative that therapists, health care workers, community organization personnel, and message designers work more closely together to address emerging challenges. These issues could include compliance with medical regimens (see Greene & Cassidy, in press), symptom management, and the need for new disease prevention strategies. Therapists could be invaluable resources for health care workers as they struggle with client compliance (and vice versa). Health care workers could, in turn, be providers of important information to public health campaign strategists. In essence, new challenges ahead could be faced more adequately if interests and knowledge of the perspectives were more closely aligned. The time for separate, field-specific work has clearly passed.

Another area where professional cross-fertilization of ideas will become important is in the development of prevention strategies. There is a fear that if the eradication agenda is promoted, HIV/AIDS prevention strategies will not be effective. Specifically, individuals might regress to past riskier behaviors once the perception of HIV/AIDS as lethal lessens. This is of particular concern because, although the level of HIV in the body can be reduced with new drug therapies, it is not totally eradicated. In fact, the terminology commonly used that HIV is reduced to "undetectable levels" is very misleading. HIV may be undetectable only because we lack sophisticated instruments to measure HIV below certain levels. It does not mean that HIV/AIDS is eliminated from the body. Therefore, not only do the general public and individuals most at risk need to be properly educated about this new era of HIV/AIDS, creative and powerful prevention efforts are still needed.

For too long, relationships of HIV-infected people have been ignored; the emphasis has been on prevention and treatment. What has been overlooked is how HIV-infected people live on a daily basis and how the infection affects their lives. The chapters in this book provide a good start in examining the social and relational consequences of HIV/AIDS. Future research on HIV/AIDS must incorporate factors such as gender and race in explaining the effects of new treatments. This is an area where more research would be especially useful. If HIV-infected people will be living longer, healthier lives, then the importance of understanding social aspects of the disease becomes even more pressing.

References

Abrams, E., & Nicholas, S. (1990). Pediatric HIV infection. *Pediatric Annals, 19,* 482-487.

Adelman, M. B. (1989). Social support and AIDS. *AIDS & Public Policy Journal, 4,* 31-39.

Adelman, M. B. (1992). Rituals of adversity and remembering: The role of possessions for persons and community living with AIDS. In J. F. Sherry, Jr. & B. Sternthal (Eds.), *Advances in consumer research* (Vol. 19, pp. 401-403). Provo, UT: Association for Consumer Research.

Adelman, M. B., & Frey, L. R. (1994). The pilgrim must embark: Creating and sustaining community in a residential facility for people with AIDS. In L. R. Frey (Ed.), *Group communication in context: Studies of natural groups* (pp. 3-22). Hillsdale, NJ: Lawrence Erlbaum.

Adelman, M. B., & Frey, L. R. (1997). *The fragile community: Living together with AIDS.* Hillsdale, NJ: Lawrence Erlbaum.

Adelman, M. B., Frey, L. R., & Budz, T. (1994). Keeping the community spirit alive. *Journal of Long-term Care Administration, 22*(2), 4-7.

Adelman, M. B. (Producer), & Schultz, P. (Director). (1991). *The pilgrim must embark: Living in community* [Videotape]. Chicago: Terra Nova Films. (Available from L. R. Frey, 744 Gordon Terrace #206, Chicago, IL 60613)

Albert, E. (1989). AIDS and the press: The creation and transformation of a social problem. In J. Best (Ed.), *Images of issues: Typifying contemporary social problems* (pp. 39-54). Hawthorne, NY: Aldine de Gruyter.

Albrecht, T. L., & Adelman, M. B. (1987a). Communicating social support: A theoretical perspective. In T. L. Albrecht, M. B. Adelman, & Associates, *Communicating social support* (pp. 18-39). Newbury Park, CA: Sage.

Albrecht, T. L., & Adelman, M. B. (1987b). Dilemmas of supportive communication. In T. L. Albrecht, M. B. Adelman, & Associates, *Communicating social support* (pp. 240-254). Newbury Park, CA: Sage.

Albrecht, T. L., Adelman, M. B., & Associates (1987c). *Communicating social support.* Newbury Park, CA: Sage.

Alloy, L. B., & Abramson, L. Y. (1979). Judgement of contingency in depressed and nondepressed students: Sadder but wiser? *Journal of Experimental Psychology: General, 108,* 441-485.

Allport, G. W. (1954). *The nature of prejudice.* Reading, MA: Addison-Wesley.

Altman, I. (1973). Reciprocity of interpersonal exchange. *Journal for Theory of Social Behavior, 3,* 249-261.

Altman, I., & Taylor, D. A. (1973). *Social penetration: The development of interpersonal relationships.* New York: Holt, Rhinehart, & Winston.

American Association for World Health. (1996). *One world one hope* [Brochure]. Washington, DC: Author.

Anderson, B., Anderson, B., & deProsse, C. (1989a). Controlled prospective longitudinal study of women with cancer. II. Psychological outcomes. *Journal of Consulting and Clinical Psychology, 57,* 692-697.

Anderson, B., Anderson, B., & deProsse, C. (1989b). Controlled prospective longitudinal study of women with cancer. I. Sexual functioning outcomes. *Journal of Consulting and Clinical Psychology, 57,* 683-691.

Antonovsky, A. (1987). *Unravelling the mystery of health: How people manage stress and stay well.* San Francisco, CA: Jossey-Bass.

Arno, P. S. (1986). The nonprofit sector's response to the AIDS epidemic: Community-based services in San Francisco. *American Journal of Public Health, 76,* 1325-1330.

Badger, T. (1990). Men with cardiovascular disease and their spouses: Coping, health, and marital adjustment. *Archives of Psychiatric Nursing, 4,* 319-324.

Badger, T. A. (1992). Coping, lifestyle changes, health perceptions, and marital adjustment in middle aged women and men with cardiovascular disease and their spouses. *Health Care for Women International, 13,* 43-55.

Barbee, A. P. (1990). Interactive coping: The cheering up process in close relationships. In S. W. Duck (Ed.), *Personal relationships and social support* (pp. 46-65). London: Sage.

Barbee, A. P., & Cunningham, M. R. (1995). An experimental approach to social support communications: Interactive coping in close relationships. In B. R. Burleson (Ed.), *Communication Yearbook 18* (pp. 381-413). Thousand Oaks, CA, Sage.

Barbee, A. P., Cunningham, M. R., Winstead, B. A., Derlega, V. J., Gulley, M. R., Yankeelov, P. A., & Druen, P. B. (1993). Effects of gender role expectations on the social support process. *Journal of Social Issues, 49*(3), 175-190.

Barrera, M., & Ainley, S. (1983). The structure of social support: A conceptual and empirical analysis. *Journal of Community Psychology, 11,* 133-143.

Bartholow, B. N., Doll, L. S., Joy, D., Douglas, J. M., Bolan, G., Harrison, J. S., Moss, P. M., & McKirnan, D. (1994). Emotional, behavioral and HIV risks associated with sexual abuse among adult homosexual and bisexual men. *Child Abuse and Neglect, 18*(9), 747-761.

Bartlett, J. G. (1996). *Medical management of HIV infection: 1996 edition.* Glenview, IL: Physicians and Scientists Publishing Co.

Barusch, A., & Spaid, W. (1989). Gender differences in caregiving: Why do wives report greater burden? *The Gerontologist, 29,* 667-676.

Baumeister, R. F., & Jones, E. E. (1978). When self-presentation is constrained by the target's knowledge: Consistency and compensation. *Journal of Personality and Social Psychology, 36,* 608-618.

Baumeister, R. F., & Leary, M. R. (1995). The need to belong: Desire for interpersonal attachments as a fundamental human motivation. *Psychological Bulletin, 117*, 497-529.

Beck, A. T. (1967). *Depression: Clinical, experimental and theoretical aspects.* New York: Harper.

Beck, A. T., & Steer, R. A. (1987). *Beck Depression Inventory: Manual.* San Antonio, TX: The Psychological Corporation, Harcourt Brace Jovanovich.

Bell, N. K. (1991). Social/sexual norms and AIDS in the South. *AIDS Education and Prevention, 3*, 164-180.

Bennett, M. J. (1990). Stigmatization: Experiences of persons with acquired immune deficiency syndrome. *Issues in Mental Health Nursing, 11*, 141-154.

Berghuis, J., & Stanton, A. (1994, August). *Infertile couples' coping and adjustment across an artificial insemination attempt.* Paper presented at the annual meeting of the American Psychological Association, Los Angeles.

Berscheid, E. (1985). Interpersonal attraction. In G. Lindzey & E. Aronson (Eds.), *The handbook of social psychology* (3rd ed., pp. 413-484). Hillsdale, NJ: Random House.

Berscheid, E., Snyder, M., & Omoto, A. M. (1989a). Issues in studying close relationships: Conceptualizing and measuring closeness. *Review of Personality and Social Psychology, 10*, 63-91.

Berscheid, E., Snyder, M., & Omoto, A. M. (1989b). The Relationship Closeness Inventory: Assessing the closeness of interpersonal relationships. *Journal of Personality and Social Psychology, 57*, 792-807.

Biddle, N., Conte, L., & Diamond, E. (1993). AIDS in the media: Entertainment or infotainment? In S. C. Ratzan (Ed.), *AIDS: Effective health communication for the 90's* (pp. 141-150). Philadelphia, PA: Taylor & Francis.

Billings, A. G., & Moos, R. H. (1981). The role of coping resources in attenuating the impact of stressful life events. *Journal of Behavioral Medicine, 4*, 157-189.

Bloom, J., & Speigel, D. (1984). The effect of two dimensions of social support on the psychological well-being and social functioning of women with advanced breast cancer. *Social Science and Medicine, 19*, 831-837.

Booth, A., & Johnson, D. (1994). Declining health and marital quality. *Journal of Marriage and the Family, 56*, 218-223.

Bouton, R. A., Gallaher, P. E., Garlinghouse, P. A., Leal, T., Rosenstein, L. D., & Young, R. K. (1987). Scales for measuring fear of AIDS and homophobia. *Journal of Personality Assessment, 51*, 606-614.

Bowman, J. M., Brown, S. T., & Eason, F. R. (1994). Attitudes of baccalaureate nursing students in one school toward acquired immune deficiency syndrome. *AIDS Education and Prevention, 6*, 535-541.

Braiker, H. B., & Kelley, H. H. (1979). Conflict in the development of close relationships. In R. L. Burgess & T. L. Huston (Eds.), *Social exchange in developing relationships.* New York: Academic Press.

Braithwaite, D. O. (1991). "Just how much did that wheelchair cost?" Management of privacy boundaries by persons with disabilities. *Western Journal of Speech Communication, 55*, 254-274.

Braithwaite, V. A. (1990). *Bound to care.* Sydney: Allen and Unwin.

Brashares, H. J., & Catanzaro, S. J. (1994). Mood regulation expectancies, coping responses, depression, and sense of burden in female caregivers of Alzheimer's patients. *Journal of Nervous and Mental Diseases, 182*(8), 437-442.

Brehm, S. S. (1992). *Intimate relationships.* New York: McGraw-Hill.

Brody, S. (1995, August). *Lying by AIDS patients and other research confounds*. Paper presented at the meeting of the American Psychological Association, New York.

Budz, T. (1993). Case management. In S. J. Miller, K. I. Ward, & R. Rybicki (Eds.), *Handbook for assisted living* (pp. 75-80). Chicago: Bonaventure House.

Burger, J. M. (1981). Motivational biases in the attribution of responsibility for an accident: A meta-analysis of the defensive-attribution hypothesis. *Psychological Bulletin, 90,* 496-512.

Burleson, B. R., Albrecht, T. L., Goldsmith, D., & Sarason, I. (1994). The communication of social support. In B. Burleson, T. Albrecht, & I. Sarason (Eds.), *Communication of social support: Messages, interactions, relationships, and community* (pp. xi-xxx). Thousand Oaks, CA: Sage.

Catania, J., Turner, H., Choi, K.-H., & Coates, T. (1992). Coping with death anxiety: Help-seeking and social support among gay men with various HIV diagnoses. *AIDS, 6,* 999-1005.

Causey, D. L., & Dubow, E. F. (1992). Development of a self report coping measure for elementary school children. *Journal of Clinical Child Psychology, 21,* 47-59.

Cawyer, C. S., & Smith-Dupré, A. (1995). Communicating social support: Identifying supportive episodes in an HIV/AIDS support group. *Communication Quarterly, 43,* 243-258.

Centers for Disease Control and Prevention. (1981). Pneumocystis pneumonia—Los Angeles. *Morbidity and Mortality Weekly Reports, 30,* 250-252.

Centers for Disease Control and Prevention. (1991, January). *HIV/AIDS Surveillance Report*. Atlanta, GA.

Centers for Disease Control and Prevention. (1992, January). *HIV/AIDS Surveillance Report*. Atlanta, GA.

Centers for Disease Control and Prevention. (1993, January). *HIV/AIDS Surveillance Report*. Atlanta, GA.

Centers for Disease Control and Prevention. (1994). *HIV/AIDS Surveillance Report, 5*(4). Atlanta, GA.

Centers for Disease Control and Prevention. (1995a). *HIV/AIDS Surveillance Report, 6*(2). Atlanta, GA.

Centers for Disease Control and Prevention. (1995b). Update: Trends in AIDS among men who have sex with men—United States, 1989-1994. *Morbidity and Mortality Weekly Reports, 44,* 401-404.

Centers for Disease Control and Prevention. (1996a). *HIV/AIDS Surveillance Report, 8*(1). Atlanta, GA.

Centers for Disease Control and Prevention. (1996b). Update: Mortality attributable to HIV infection among persons aged 25-44 years—United States, 1994. *Morbidity and Mortality Weekly Report, 45,* 121-125.

Centers for Disease Control and Prevention. (1996c). *HIV/AIDS surveillance report, 8*(2). Atlanta, GA.

Centers for Disease Control and Prevention. (1997). *HIV/AIDS Surveillance Report, 9*(1), Atlanta, GA.

Chambré, S. (1989). Kindling points of light: Volunteering as public policy. *Nonprofit and Voluntary Sector Quarterly, 20,* 267-288.

Chambré, S. M. (1991). The volunteer response to the AIDS epidemic in New York City: Implications for research on volunteerism. *Nonprofit and Voluntary Sector Quarterly, 20,* 267-287.

Chan, C. (1993). Issues of identity development among Asian-American lesbians and gay men. In L. D. Garnets & D. C. Kimmel (Eds.), *Psychological perspectives on lesbian and gay male experiences* (pp. 376-388). New York: Columbia University Press.

Chan, C. (1995). Issues of sexual identity in an ethnic minority: The case of Chinese American lesbians, gay men, and bisexual people. In A. R. D'Augelli & C. J. Patterson (Eds.), *Lesbian, gay and bisexual identities over the lifespan* (pp. 87-101). New York: Oxford University Press.

Cherry, K., & Smith, D. H. (1993). Sometimes I cry: The experience of loneliness for men with AIDS. *Health Communication, 5,* 181-208.

Chesney, M., & Folkman, S. (1994). Psychological impact of HIV disease and implications for intervention. *Psychiatric Manifestations of HIV Disease, 17*(1), 163-182.

Christ, G. H., Wiener, L. S., & Moynihan, R. T. (1986). Psychosocial issues in AIDS. *Psychiatric Annals, 16,* 173, 175.

Clark, M. S. (1983). Some implications of close social bonds for help-seeking. In B. M. DePaulo, A. Nadler, & J. D. Fisher (Eds.), *New directions in helping: Vol. 2. Help-seeking* (pp. 205-229). New York: Academic Press.

Coates, D., Renzagla, G. J., & Embree, M. C. (1983). When helping backfires: Help and helplessness. In B. M. DePaulo, A. Nadler, & J. D. Fisher (Eds.), *New directions in helping: Vol. 2. Help-seeking* (pp. 251-279). New York: Academic Press.

Coates, D., & Winston, T. (1983). Counteracting the deviance of depression: Peer support groups for victims. *Journal of Social Issues, 39*(2), 169-194.

Cobb, S. (1976). Social support as a moderator of life stress. *Psychosomatic Medicine, 38,* 300-314.

Cohen, J., & Cohen, P. (1983). *Applied multiple regression/correlation analysis for the behavioral sciences* (2nd ed.). Hillsdale, NJ: Lawrence Erlbaum.

Cohen, S., & Wills, T. A. (1985). Stress, social support, and the buffering hypothesis. *Psychological Bulletin, 98,* 310-357.

Collins, R. L. (1994). Social support provision to HIV-infected gay men. *Journal of Applied Social Psychology, 24,* 1848-1869.

Collins, R. L., & Di Paula, A. (1997). Personality and the provision of support: Emotions felt and signaled. In G. Pierce, B. Lakey, I. G. Sarason, & B. Sarason (Eds.), *Sourcebook of theory and research on social support and personality* (pp. 429-443). New York: Plenum.

Collins, R. L., Taylor, S. E., & Skokan, L. A. (1990). A better world or a shattered vision? Changes in life perspectives following victimization. *Social Cognition, 8,* 263-285.

Coopersmith, S. (1967). *The antecedents of self-esteem.* San Francisco, CA: W. H. Freeman.

Coyne, J., & Smith, D. (1991). Couples coping with a myocardial infarction: Contextual perspective on wives' distress. *Journal of Personality and Social Psychology, 61,* 404-412.

Coyne, J. C., Ellard, J. H., & Smith, D. A. F. (1990). Social support, interdependence, and the dilemmas of helping. In B. R. Sarason, I. G. Sarason, & G. R. Pierce (Eds.), *Social Support: An interactional view* (pp. 129-149). New York: Wiley.

Crandall, C. S., & Coleman, R. (1992). AIDS-related stigmatization and the disruption of social relationships. *Journal of Social and Personal Relationships, 9,* 163-177.

Crawford, A. M. (1996). Stigma associated with AIDS: A meta-analysis. *Journal of Applied Social Psychology, 26,* 398-416.

Crawford, R. (1994). The boundaries of the self and the unhealthy other: Reflections on health, culture, and AIDS. *Social Science and Medicine, 10,* 1347-1365.

Crocker, J., & Major, B. (1989). Social stigma and self-esteem: The self-protective properties of stigma. *Psychological Review, 96,* 608-630.

Cronkite, R. C., & Moos, R. H. (1984). The role of predisposing and moderating factors in the stress-illness relationship. *Journal of Health and Social Behavior, 25,* 372-393.

Cunningham, J. A., Strassberg, D. S., & Haas, B. (1986). Effects of intimacy and sex-role congruency on self-disclosure. *Journal of Social and Clinical Psychology, 4,* 393-401.

Dakof, G. A., & Taylor, S. E. (1990). Victim's perceptions of social support: What is helpful from whom? *Journal of Personality and Social Psychology, 58,* 80-89.

Dane, B. O., & Miller, S. O. (1992). *AIDS: Intervening with hidden grievers.* Westport, CT: Auburn House.

Daniolos, P. T. (1994). House calls: A support group for individuals with AIDS in a community residential setting. *International Journal of Group Psychotherapy, 44,* 133-152.

Davis, F. (1961). Deviance disavowal: The management of strained interaction by the visibly handicapped. *Social Problems, 9,* 120-132.

Davis, M. (1993, August 30). Patient sues after workers view diagnosis. *Virginian-Pilot,* pp. D1, D4.

Dawson, D. A., Cynamon, M., & Fitti, J. E. (1987). AIDS knowledge and attitudes: Provisional data from the national health interview survey. *Advancedata, 146,* 1-10.

Dean, A., & Lin, N. (1977). The stress-buffering role of social support. *Journal of Nervous and Mental Disease, 165,* 403-417.

Deaux, K., Wrightsman, L. S., Sigelman, C. K., & Sundstrom, E. (1988). *Social psychology.* Pacific Grove, CA: Brooks/Cole.

Debats, D. L. (1996). Meaning in life: Clinical relevance and predictive power. *British Journal of Clinical Psychology, 35,* 503-516.

DeJong, W. (1980). The stigma of obesity: The consequences of naive assumptions concerning the causes of physical deviance. *Journal of Health and Social Behavior, 21,* 75-87.

DeMarco, J. (1983). Gay racism. In M. J. Smith (Ed.), *Black men/white men: A gay anthology* (pp. 109-118). San Francisco, CA: Gay Sunshine Press.

Derlega, V. J., Metts, S., Petronio, S., & Margulis, S. T. (1993). *Self-disclosure.* Newbury Park, CA: Sage.

Derogatis, L. (1977). *SCL-90 manual.* Baltimore, MD: Clinical Psychometric Research.

Dew, A., Ragni, M., & Nimorwicz, P. (1990). Infection with human immunodeficiency virus and vulnerability to psychiatric distress. *Archives of General Psychiatry, 47,* 737-744.

DiDomenico, M. J. (1993). Pastoral care at Bonaventure House. In S. J. Miller, K. I. Ward, & R. Rybicki (Eds.), *Handbook for assisted living* (pp. 111-120). Chicago: Bonaventure House.

Donlou, J. N., Wolcott, D. L., Gottlieb, M. S., & Landsverk, J. (1985). Psychosocial aspects of AIDS and AIDS-related complex: A pilot study. *Journal of Psychosocial Oncology, 3,* 39-55.

Dworkin, S. H., & Pincu, L. (1993). Counseling in the era of AIDS. *Journal of Counseling and Development, 71,* 275-281.

Edgar, T., Fitzpatrick, M. A., & Freimuth, V. S. (Eds.). (1992). *AIDS: A communication perspective.* Hillsdale, NJ: Lawrence Erlbaum.

Ekberg, J., Griffith, N., & Foxall, M. (1986). Spouse burnout syndrome. *Journal of Advanced Nursing, 11,* 161-165.

Elliot, D., Trief, P., & Stein, N. (1986). Mastery, stress, and coping in marriage among chronic pain patients. *Journal of Behavioral Medicine, 9,* 549-558.

Elliott, G. C., Ziegler, H. L., Altman, B. M., & Scott, D. R. (1982). Understanding stigma: Dimensions of deviance and coping. *Deviant Behavior, 3,* 275-300.

Espin, O. (1993). Issues of identity in the psychology of Latina lesbians. In L. D. Garnets & D. C. Kimmel (Eds.), *Psychological perspectives on lesbian and gay male experiences* (pp. 348-363). New York: Columbia University Press.

Evans, D. L., Leserman, J., Perkins, D. O., Stern, R. A., Murphy, C., Zheng, B., Gattes, D., Longmate, J. A., Silva, S. G., van der Horst, C. M., Hall, C. D., Folds, J. D., Golden, R. N., & Petitto, J. M. (1997). Severe life stress as a predictor of early disease progression in HIV infection. *American Journal of Psychiatry, 154,* 630-774.

Fanos, J., & Wiener, L. (1994). Tomorrow's survivors: Siblings of human immunodeficiency virus-infected children. *Behavioral and Developmental Pediatrics, 15,* S43-S48.

Farina, A., Holland, C. H., & Ring, K. (1966). The role of stigma and set in interpersonal interaction. *Journal of Abnormal Psychology, 70,* 47-51.

Farina, A., Wheeler, D. S., & Mehta, S. (1991). The impact of an unpleasant and demeaning social interaction. *Journal of Social and Clinical Psychology, 10,* 351-371.

Fehr, B. (1996). *Friendship processes.* Thousand Oaks, CA: Sage.

Finkelstein, F. O., Finkelstein, S. H., & Steele, T. E. (1976). Assessment of marital relationships of hemodialysis clients. *American Journal of Medical Science, 271,* 21-28.

Fish, R. A., & Rye, B. J. (1991). Attitudes toward a homosexual or heterosexual with AIDS. *Journal of Applied Social Psychology, 21,* 651-667.

Fitting, M., Rabins, P., Lucas, M., & Eastham, J. (1986). Caregivers for dementia patients: A comparison of husbands and wives. *The Gerontologist, 26,* 248-259.

Flor, H., Turk, D., & Rudy, T. (1987). Pain and families. II. Assessment and treatment. *Pain, 30,* 29-45.

Folkman, S. (1984). Personal control and stress and coping processes: A theoretical analysis. *Journal of Personality and Social Psychology, 46,* 839-852.

Folkman, S. (1993). Psychosocial effects of HIV infection. In L. Goldberger & S. Breznitz (Eds.), *Handbook of stress* (2nd ed., pp. 658-681). New York: Free Press.

Folkman, S. (1997, July). *Caregivers of persons with AIDS.* Paper presented at the fifth annual research conference on the "Role of Families in Preventing and Adapting to HIV/AIDS," sponsored by the Office on AIDS, National Institute of Mental Health, Baltimore, MD.

Folkman, S., Chesney, M. A., & Christopher-Richards, A. (1994). Stress and coping in caregiving partners of men with AIDS. *Psychiatric Manifestations of HIV Disease, 17,* 35-53.

Folkman, S., Chesney, M., Pollack, L., & Coates, T. (1993). Stress, control, coping and depressive mood in human immunodeficiency virus-positive and -negative gay men in San Francisco. *Journal of Nervous and Mental Diseases, 181,* 409-416.

Folkman, S., & Lazarus, R. (1980). An analysis of coping in a middle-aged community sample. *Journal of Health and Social Behavior, 21,* 219-239.

Folkman, S., Lazarus, R. S., Dunkel-Schetter, C., DeLongis, A., & Gruen, R. (1986). Dynamics of a stressful encounter: Cognitive appraisal, coping, and encounter outcomes. *Journal of Personality and Social Psychology, 50,* 992-1003.

Frable, D. E. S., Blackstone, T., & Scherbaum, C. (1990). Marginal and mindful: Deviants in social interactions. *Journal of Personality and Social Psychology, 59,* 140-149.

Frankl, V. (1984). *Man's search for meaning.* New York: Washington Square Press.

Freimuth, V. S., Hammond, S. L., Edgar, T., & Monahan, J. L. (1990). Reaching those at risk: A content-analytic study of AIDS PSAs. *Communication Research, 17,* 775-791.

Frey, L. R. (1994). The naturalistic paradigm: Studying small groups in the postmodern era. *Small Group Research, 25,* 551-577.

Frey, L. R., & Adelman, M. B. (1993). Building community life: Understanding individual, group, and organizational processes. In S. J. Miller, K. I. Ward, & R. Rybicki (Eds.), *Handbook for assisted living* (pp. 31-40). Chicago: Bonaventure House.

Frey, L. R., Adelman, M. B., & Query, J. L., Jr. (1996). Communication practices in the social construction of health in an AIDS residence. *Journal of Health Psychology, 1,* 383-397.

Fullerton, C. S., McCarroll, J. E., Ursano, R. J., & Wright, K. M. (1992). Psychological responses of rescue workers: Fire fighters and trauma. *American Journal of Psychosocial Oncology, 62,* 371-378.

Fullilove, M. T. (1989). Anxiety and stigmatizing aspects of HIV infection. *Journal of Clinical Psychiatry, 50,* 5-8.

Fullilove, M. T., Fullilove, R. E., Haynes, K., & Gross, S. (1990). Black women and AIDS prevention: A view towards understanding the gender rules. *Journal of Sex Research, 27,* 47-64.

Geballe, S., Gruendel, J., & Andiman, W. (Eds.). (1995). *Forgotten children of the AIDS epidemic.* New Haven, CT: Yale University Press.

Gingrich answers attack on AIDS research. (1995, July 6). *Winston-Salem Journal,* p. B3.

Glass, R. M. (1988). AIDS and suicide. *Journal of the American Medical Association, 259,* 1369-1370.

Goffman, E. (1963). *Stigma: Notes on the management of spoiled identity.* Englewood Cliffs, NJ: Prentice Hall.

Goldsmith, D. (1992). Managing conflicting goals in supportive interaction: An integrative theoretical framework. *Communication Research, 19,* 264-286.

Goldsmith, D. (1994). The role of facework in supportive communication. In B. R. Burleson, T. L. Albrecht, & I. G. Sarason (Eds.), *Communication of social support: Messages, interactions, relationships, and community* (pp. 29-49). Thousand Oaks, CA: Sage.

Gove, W., Hughes, M., & Style, C. (1983). Does marriage have positive effects on the well-being of the individual? *Journal of Health and Social Behavior, 24,* 122-131.

Greenberg, M. A., & Stone, A. A. (1992). Emotional disclosure about traumas and its relation to health: Effects of previous disclosure and trauma severity. *Journal of Personality and Social Psychology, 63,* 75-84.

Greenblatt, M., Becerra, R. M., & Serafetinides, E. A. (1982). Social networks and mental health: An overview. *American Journal of Psychiatry, 139,* 977-984.

Greene, K., & Cassidy, B. J. (in press). Ethical choices regarding noncompliance: Prescribing protease inhibitors for HIV infected adolescent females. In W. N. Elwood (Ed.), *Power in the blood: AIDS, politics, and communication.* Hillsdale, NJ: Lawrence Erlbaum.

Greene, K., & Serovich, J. M. (1996). Appropriateness of disclosure of HIV testing information: The perspective of PLWAs. *Journal of Applied Communication Research, 24,* 50-65.

Greif, G. L., & Porembski, E. (1988). AIDS and significant others: Findings from a preliminary exploration of needs. *Health and Social Work, 13,* 259-265.

Guinan, J., McCallum, L., Painter, L., & Dykes, J. (1991). Stressors and rewards of being an AIDS emotional-support volunteer: A scale for use by care-givers for people with AIDS. *AIDS Care, 3,* 137-150.

Gulley, M. R. (1993). *Sequential analyses of social support elicitation and provision behaviors.* Unpublished doctoral dissertation, University of Louisville.

Gussow, Z., & Tracy, G. S. (1968). Status, ideology, and adaptation to stigmatized illness: A study of leprosy. *Human Organization, 27,* 316-325.

Hallett, M. A., & Cannella, D. (1994). Gatekeeping through media format: Strategies of voice for the HIV-positive via human interest news formats and organizations. *Journal of Homosexuality, 26,* 111-134.

Harter, S. (1985). *Manual for the Self-Perception Profile for Children.* Denver, CO: University of Denver.

Harter, S. (1988). *Manual for the Self-Perception Profile for Adolescents.* Denver, CO: University of Denver.

Haverkos, H. W., & Quinn, T. C. (1995). The third wave: HIV infection among heterosexuals in the United States and Europe. *International Journal of STD and AIDS, 6*(4), 227-232.

Hays, R. B., Catania, J. A., McKusick, L., & Coates, T. J. (1990). Help-seeking for AIDS-related concerns: A comparison of gay men with various HIV diagnoses. *American Journal of Community Psychology, 18,* 743-755.

Hays, R. B., Chauncey, S., & Tobey, L. A. (1990). The social support networks of gay men with AIDS. *Journal of Community Psychology, 18,* 374-385.

Hays, R. B., McKusick, L., Pollack, L., Hilliard, R., Hoff, C., & Coates, T. J. (1993). Disclosing HIV seropositivity to significant others. *AIDS, 7,* 425-431.

Hays, R. B., Turner, H., & Coates, T. J. (1992). Social support, AIDS-related symptoms, and depression among gay men. *Journal of Consulting and Clinical Psychology, 60,* 463-469.

Helgeson, V. S. (1991). The effects of masculinity and social support on recovery from myocardial infarction. *Psychosomatic Medicine, 53,* 621-633.

Hellinger, F. J. (1993). The lifetime cost of treating a person with HIV. *Journal of the American Medical Association, 270,* 474-478.

Herek, G. M. (1990a). The context of anti-gay violence: Notes on cultural and psychological heterosexism. *Journal of Interpersonal Violence, 5,* 316-333.

Herek, G. M. (1990b). Illness, stigma, and AIDS. In P. Costa & G. R. VandenBos (Eds.), *Psychological aspects of serious illness* (pp. 107-149). Washington, DC: American Psychological Association.

Herek, G. M., & Capitanio, J. P. (1993). Public reactions to AIDS in the United States: A second decade of stigma. *American Journal of Public Health, 83,* 574-577.

Herek, G. M., & Glunt, E. K. (1988). An epidemic of stigma: Public reactions to AIDS. *American Psychologist, 43,* 886-891.

Herek, G. M., & Glunt, E. K. (1995). Identity and community among gay and bisexual men in the AIDS era: Preliminary findings from the Sacramento Men's Health Study. In G. M. Herek & B. Greene (Eds.), *AIDS, identity, and community: The HIV epidemic and lesbians and gay men* (pp. 55-83). Thousand Oaks: Sage.

Herek, G. M., & Greene, B. (Eds.). (1995). *AIDS, identity, and community: The HIV epidemic and lesbians and gay men.* Thousand Oaks, CA: Sage.

Herman, N. J. (1993). Return to sender: Reintegrative stigma-management strategies of ex-psychiatric patients. *Journal of Contemporary Ethnography, 22,* 295-330.

Hiller, D. V. (1982). Overweight as a master status: A replication. *Journal of Psychology, 110,* 107-113.

Hobfoll, S. E., & London, P. (1986). The relationship of self-concept and social support to emotional distress among women during war. *Journal of Social and Clinical Psychology, 4,* 189-203.

Hoff, C. C., McKusick, L., Hilliard, B., & Coates, T. J. (1992). The impact of HIV antibody status on gay men's partner preferences: A community perspective. *AIDS Education and Prevention, 4,* 197-204.

Hoffman, M. A. (1991). Counseling the HIV-infected client: A psychological assessment and intervention. *Counseling Psychologist, 19,* 467-542.

Hoffman, M. A. (1996). *Counseling clients with HIV disease: Assessment, intervention, and prevention.* New York: Guilford.

Holahan, C. J., & Moos, R. H. (1987). Risk, resistance, and psychological distress: A longitudinal analysis with adults and children. *Journal of Abnormal Psychology, 96*, 3-13.

Holmberg, S. D. (1996). The estimated prevalence and incidence of HIV in 96 large US metropolitan areas. *American Journal of Public Health, 86*, 642-654.

Horowitz, M. J. (1979). Psychological responses to serious life events. In V. Hamilton & D. M. Warburton (Eds.), *Human stress and cognition: An information processing approach* (pp. 237-265). Chichester, England: Wiley.

House, J. S., Landis, K. R., & Umberson, D. (1988). Social relationships and health. *Science, 241*, 540-545.

Hurt, H. T. (1989, May). *The relationships among interpersonal skills, social support, and recovery from alcohol addiction.* Paper presented at the meeting of the International Communication Association, San Francisco, CA.

Huszti, H. C., Clopton, J. R., & Mason, P. J. (1989). Acquired immune deficiency syndrome educational program: Effects on adolescents' knowledge and attitudes. *Pediatrics, 84*, 986-994.

Icard, L. (1986). Black gay men and conflicting social identities: Sexual orientation versus racial identity. *Journal of Social Work and Human Sexuality: Social work practice in sexual problems, 4*(1/2), 83-93.

Ickovics, J., & Rodin, J. (1992). Women and AIDS in the United States: Epidemiology, natural history and mediating mechanisms. *Health Psychology, 11*, 1-16.

Jackson, J. S., Neighbors, H. W., & Gurin, G. (1986). Findings from a national survey of Black mental health: Implications for practice and training. In M. R. Miranda & H. H. Kitano (Eds.), *Mental health research in minority communities* (pp. 91-116). Rockville, MD: National Institutes of Mental Health.

Jacobsen, P., Perry, S., & Hirsch, D. (1990). Behavioral and psychological responses to HIV antibody testing. *Journal of Consulting and Clinical Psychology, 58*, 31-37.

Janoff-Bulman, R. (1989). Assumptive worlds and the stress of traumatic events: Applications of the schema construct. *Social Cognition, 7*, 113-136.

Janoff-Bulman, R. (1992). *Shattered assumptions: Towards a new psychology of trauma.* New York: Free Press.

Janoff-Bulman, R., & Frieze, I. H. (1983). A theoretical perspective for understanding reactions to victimization. *Journal of Social Issues, 39*, 1-17.

Jenkins, R. A. (1995). Religion and HIV: Implications for research and intervention. *Journal of Social Issues, 51*, 131-144.

Johnson, S. D. (1987). Factors related to the intolerance of AIDS victims. *Journal of the Scientific Study of Religion, 26*, 105-110.

Johnston, D., Stall, R., & Smith, K. (1995). Reliance by gay men and intravenous drug users on friends and family for AIDS-related care. *AIDS Care, 7*, 307-319.

Jones, E. E., Farina, A., Hastorf, A. H., Markus, H., Miller, D. T., & Scott, R. A. (1984). *Social stigma: The psychology of marked relationships.* New York: W. H. Freeman.

Jourard, S. M. (1972). *The transparent self.* Princeton, NJ: Van Nostrand.

Joyce, M. (1997, July 15). AIDS deaths drop by 19 percent. *Virginian-Pilot*, pp. A1, A12.

Kahn, J. O., & Hecht, F. (1996, December). Treating primary infection: Does early intervention alter the course of HIV disease? *HIV Newsline, 2*, 135-142.

Kaisch, K., & Anton-Culver, H. (1989). Psychological and social consequences of HIV exposure: Homosexuals in Southern California. *Psychology and Health, 3*, 63-75.

Kalichman, S. C. (1995). *Understanding AIDS: A guide for mental health professionals.* Washington, DC: American Psychological Association.

Kamenga, M., Ryder, R., Jingu, M., Mbuyi, N., Mbu, L., Behets, F., Brown, C., & Heyward, W. (1990). Evidence of marked sexual behavior change associated with low HIV-1 seroconversion in 149 married couples with discordant HIV-1 serostatus: Experience at an HIV counseling center in Zaire. *AIDS, 5*, 61-67.

Kayal, P. M. (1993). *Bearing witness: Gay men's health crisis and the politics of AIDS.* Boulder, CO: Westview.

Kelley, H. H., Berscheid, E., Christensen, A., Harvey, J. H., Huston, T. L., Levinger, G., McClintock, E., Peplau, L. A., & Peterson, D. R. (1983). *Close relationships.* New York: W. H. Freeman.

Kelly, J., & Sykes, P. (1989). Helping the helpers: A support group for family members of persons with AIDS. *Social Work, 34,* 239-242.

Kelly, J. A. (1995). *Changing HIV risk behavior: Practical strategies.* New York: Guilford.

Kelly, J. A., Murphy, D. A., Bahr, R., Koob, J. J., Morgan, M. G., Kalichman, S. C., Stevenson, L. Y., Barsfield, T. L., Bernstein, B. M., & St. Lawrence, S. S. (1993). Factors associated with severity of depression and high-risk sexual behavior among persons diagnosed with HIV infection. *Health Psychology, 12,* 215-219.

Kelly, J. A., St. Lawrence, J. S., Smith, S., Jr., Hood, H. V., & Cook, D. J. (1987a). Medical students' attitudes toward AIDS and homosexual patients. *Journal of Medical Education, 62, 549-556.*

Kelly, J. A., St. Lawrence, J. S., Smith, S., Jr., Hood, H. V., & Cook, D. J. (1987b). Stigmatization of AIDS patients by physicians. *American Journal of Public Health, 77,* 789-791.

Kelly, J. J., Chu, S. Y., & Buehler, J. W. (1993). AIDS deaths shift from hospital to home. *American Journal of Public Health, 83,* 1433-1437.

Kemeny, M. E., Weiner, H., Taylor, S. E., Schneider, S., Visscher, B., & Fahey, J. L. (1994). Repeated bereavement, depressed mood, and immune parameters in HIV seropositive and seronegative gay men. *Health Psychology, 13*(1), 14-24.

Kenny, D. A. (1988). The analysis of data from two-person relationships. In S. W. Duck (Ed.), *Handbook of personal relationships* (pp. 57-77). New York: John Wiley.

Kessler, R. C., & McLeod, J. D. (1985). Social support and mental health in community samples. In S. Cohen and S. L. Syme (Eds.), *Social support and health* (pp. 219-240). New York: Academic Press.

Kimberly, J. A., Serovich, J. M., & Greene, K. (1995). Disclosure of HIV-positive status: Five women's stories. *Family Relations, 44,* 316-322.

King, M. (1989). Psychological status of 192 outpatients with HIV infection and AIDS. *British Journal of Psychiatry, 154,* 237-242.

Kite, M. E., & Whitley, B. E., Jr. (1996). Sex differences in attitudes toward homosexual persons, behaviors, and civil rights: A meta-analysis. *Personality and Social Psychology Bulletin, 22,* 336-353.

Klein, K., Forehand, R., Armistead, L., & Wierson, M. (1994). The contributions of social support and coping methods to stress resiliency in couples facing hemophilia and HIV. *Advanced Behavior Research Therapy, 16,* 1-23.

Klimes, I., Catalan, J., Garrod, A., Day, A., Bond, A., & Rizza, C. (1992). Partners of men with HIV infection and hemophilia: Controlled investigation of factors associated with psychological morbidity. *AIDS Care, 4*(2), 149-156.

Klonoff, E., & Ewers, D. (1990). Care of AIDS patients as a source of stress to nursing staff. *AIDS Education and Prevention, 2,* 338-348.

Kotchick, B., Forehand, R., Armistead, L., Klein, K., & Wierson, M. (1996). Coping with illness: Interrelationships across family members and predictors of psychological adjustment. *Journal of Family Planning, 10*(3), 358-370.

Kurdek, L. A., & Schmitt, J. P. (1987). Perceived emotional support from family and friends in members of homosexual, married, and heterosexual cohabiting couples. *Journal of Homosexuality, 14*(3/4), 57-68.

Lackner, J. B., Joseph, J. G., Ostrow, D. G., Kessler, R. C., Eshleman, S., Wortman, C. B., O'Brien, K., Phair, J. P., & Chmiel, J. (1993). A longitudinal study of psychological distress in a cohort of gay men: Effects of social support and coping strategies. *Journal of Nervous and Mental Disease, 181*, 4-12.

La Gaipa, J. J. (1990). The negative effects of informal support systems. In S. W. Duck (Ed., with R. C. Silber), *Personal relationships and social support* (pp. 122-139). London: Sage.

Lane, J. D., & Wegner, D. M. (1995). The cognitive consequences of secrecy. *Journal of Personality and Social Psychology, 69*, 237-253.

Lang-Takac, E., & Osterweil, Z. (1992). Separateness and connectedness: Differences between the genders. *Sex Roles, 27*, 277-289.

Larson, D. G., & Chastain, R. L. (1990). Self-concealment: Conceptualization, measurement, and health implications. *Journal of Social and Clinical Psychology, 9*, 439-455.

Leary, M. R., & Downs, D. L. (1995). Interpersonal functions of the self-esteem motive: The self-esteem system as a sociometer. In M. Kernis (Ed.), *Efficacy, agency, and self-esteem* (pp. 123-144). New York: Plenum.

Leary, M. R., & Kowalski, R. M. (1995). *Social anxiety*. New York: Guilford.

Leary, M. R., Tambor, E. S., Terdal, S. J., & Downs, D. L. (1995). Self-esteem as an interpersonal monitor: The sociometer hypothesis. *Journal of Personality and Social Psychology, 68*, 518-530.

Lebowitz, L., & Roth, S. (1990, October). *The sociocultural context and women's response to being raped.* Paper presented at the International Society for Traumatic Stress, New Orleans.

Lehman, D. R., Ellard, J. H., & Wortman, C. B. (1986). Social support for the bereaved: Recipients' and providers' perspectives on what is helpful. *Journal of Consulting and Clinical Psychology, 54*, 438-446.

Leiber, L., Plumb, M. M., Gerstenzang, M. L., & Holland, J. (1976). The communication of affection between cancer patients and their spouses. *Psychosomatic Medicine, 38*, 379-389.

Leland, J. (1996, December 2). The end of AIDS? *Newsweek*, 64-68, 71, 73.

Lerner, M. J. (1970). The desire for justice and reactions to victims. In J. Macaulay & L. Berkowitz (Eds.), *Altruism and helping behavior* (pp. 205-229). New York: Academic Press.

Lerner, M. J. (1980). *The belief in a just world: A fundamental delusion.* New York: Plenum.

Lerner, M. J., & Miller, D. T. (1978). Just world research and the attribution process: Looking back and ahead. *Psychological Bulletin, 85*, 1031-1051.

Leserman, J., Perkins, D. O., & Evans, D. L. (1992). Coping with the threat of AIDS: The role of social support. *American Journal of Psychiatry, 149*, 1514-1520.

Leserman, J., DiSantostefano, R., Perkins, D. O., & Evans, D. L. (1994). Gay identification and psychological health in HIV-positive and HIV-negative gay men. *Journal of Applied Social Psychology, 24*, 2193-2208.

Levin, B. W., Krantz, D. H., Driscoll, J. M., & Fleischman, A. R. (1995). The treatment of non-HIV-related conditions in newborns at risk for HIV: A survey of neonatologists. *American Journal of Public Health, 85*, 1507-1513.

Levin, L. S., & Idler, E. I. (1981). *The hidden health care system: Mediating structures and medicine.* Cambridge, MA: Ballinger.

Levine, J. M., & McBurney, D. H. (1977). Causes and consequences of effluvia: Body odor awareness and controllability as determinants of interpersonal evaluation. *Personality and Social Psychology Bulletin, 3,* 442-445.

Levine, M. P. (1992). The life and death of gay clones. In G. Herdt (Ed.), *Gay culture in America: Essays from the field* (pp. 68-86). Boston: Beacon.

Lewis, F., Woods, N., Hough, E., & Bensley, L. (1989). The family's functioning with chronic illness in the mother: The spouse's perspective. *Social Science and Medicine, 29,* 1261-1269.

Lewis, L. S., & Range, L. M. (1992). Do means of transmission, risk knowledge, and gender affect AIDS stigma and social interactions? *Journal of Social Behavior and Personality, 7,* 211-216.

Libow, J. (1992). Traumatized children and the news media: Clinical considerations. *American Journal of Orthopsychiatry, 62,* 379-386.

Lichtman, R., & Taylor, S. (1986). Close relationships and the female cancer patient. In B. L. Anderson (Ed.), *Women with cancer: Psychological perspectives* (pp. 233-256). New York: Springer-Verlag.

Lichtman, R., Taylor, S., & Wood, J. (1987). Social support and marital adjustment after breast cancer. *Journal of Psychosocial Oncology, 5*(3), 47-76.

Lifson, A. R., Hessol, N. A., & Rutherford, G. W. (1992). Progression and clinical outcome of infection due to human immunodeficiency virus. *Clinical Infectious Diseases, 14,* 966-971.

Limandri, B. J. (1989). Disclosure of stigmatizing conditions: The discloser's perspective. *Archives of Psychiatric Nursing, 3,* 69-78.

Link, R. N., Feingold, A. R., Charap, M. H., Freeman, K., & Shelov, S. P. (1988). Concerns of medical and pediatric house officers about acquiring AIDS from their patients. *American Journal of Public Health, 78,* 455-459.

Lippmann, S., James, W., & Frierson, R. (1993). AIDS and the family: Implications for counseling. *AIDS Care, 5,* 71-78.

Lipson, M. (1993). What do you say to a child with AIDS? *Hastings Center Report, 23,* 6-12.

Loewy, E. H. (1986). AIDS and the physician's fear of contagion. *Chest, 89,* 325-326.

Loiacano, D. K. (1993). Gay identity issues among Black Americans: Racism, homophobia, and the need for validation. In L. D. Garnets & D. C. Kimmel (Eds.), *Psychological perspectives on lesbian and gay male experiences* (pp. 364-375). New York: Columbia University Press.

Lorenson, M. (1985). Effects on elderly women's self-care in case of acute hospitalization as compared with men. *Health Care for Women International, 6,* 247-265.

Maguire, G. P., Lee, E. G., Bevington, D. J., Kuchemann, C. S., Crabtree, R. J., & Cornell, C. E. (1978). Psychiatric problems in the first year after mastectomy. *British Medical Journal, 1,* 963-965.

Maione, M., & McKee, J. (1987). AIDS: Implications for counselors. *Journal of Humanistic Education and Development, 26,* 12-23.

Manne, S. L., & Zautra, A. J. (1989). Spouse criticism and support: Their association with coping and psychological adjustment among women with rheumatoid arthritis. *Journal of Personality and Social Psychology, 56*(4), 608-617.

Manne, S. L., & Zautra, A. J. (1990). Couples coping with chronic illness: Women with rheumatoid arthritis and their healthy husbands. *Journal of Behavioral Medicine, 13*(4), 327-342.

Marin, G. (1989). AIDS prevention among Hispanics: Needs, risk behaviors, and cultural values. *Public Health Reports, 104,* 411-415.

Marks, G., Bundek, N. I., Richardson, J. L., Ruiz, M. S., Maldonado, N., & Mason, H.R.C. (1992). Self-disclosure of HIV infection: Preliminary results from a sample of Hispanic men. *Health Psychology, 11*, 300-306.

Marks, G., Richardson, J. L., Ruiz, M. S., & Maldonado, N. (1992). HIV-infected men's practices in notifying past sexual partners of infection risk. *Public Health Reports, 107*, 100-105.

Martin, J. L. (1988). Psychological consequences of AIDS-related bereavement among gay men. *Journal of Consulting and Clinical Psychology, 56*(4), 856-862.

Marzuk, P. M., Tierney, H., Tardiff, K., Gross, E. M., Morgan, E., Hsu, M., & Mann, J. (1988). Increased risk of suicide in persons with AIDS. *Journal of the American Medical Association, 259*, 1333-1337.

Mason, H. R. C., Marks, G., Simoni, J. M., Ruiz, M. S., & Richardson, J. L. (1995). Culturally sanctioned secrets? Latino men's nondisclosure of HIV infection to family, friends, and lovers. *Health Psychology, 14*, 6-12.

Mays, V. M., Cochran, S. D., & Bellinger, G. (1992, June). *Factors influencing AIDS risk perception of Black gay men.* Paper presented at the 8th International Conference on AIDS, Amsterdam.

Mays, V. M., Cochran, S. D., & Rhue, S. (1993). The impact of perceived discrimination on the interpersonal relationships of Black lesbians. *Journal of Homosexuality, 25*, 1-14.

McAllister, M. P. (1992). AIDS, medicalization, and the news media. In T. Edgar, M. A. Fitzpatrick, & V. S. Freimuth (Eds.), *AIDS: A communication perspective* (pp. 195-221). Hillsdale, NJ: Lawrence Erlbaum.

McCain, N. L., & Gramling, L. F. (1992). Living with dying: Coping with HIV disease. *Issues in Mental Health Nursing, 13*, 271-284.

McCann, I. L., & Pearlman, L. (1990). *Through a glass darkly: Understanding and treating the adult trauma survivor through constructivist self development theory.* New York: Brunner/Mazel.

McCann, I. L., Sakheim, D. K., & Abrahamson, D. J. (1988). Trauma and victimization: A model of psychological adaptation. *Counseling Psychologist, 16*(4), 531-594.

McCann, K., & Wadsworth, E. (1992). The role of informal carers in supporting gay men who have HIV related illness: What do they do and what are their needs? *AIDS Care, 4*, 25-34.

McKirnan, D., Ostrow, D., & Hope, B. (1996). Sex, drugs, and escape: A psychological model of HIV-risk sexual behaviours. *AIDS Care, 8*, 655-669.

Mehta, S. I., & Farina, A. (1988). Associative stigma: Perceptions of the difficulties of college-aged children of stigmatized fathers. *Journal of Social and Clinical Psychology, 7*, 192-202.

Memon, A. (1990). Young people's knowledge, beliefs and attitudes about HIV/AIDS: A review of research. *Health Education Research, 5*, 327-335.

Metts, S., Manns, H., & Kruzic, L. (1996). Social support structures and predictors of depression in persons who are seropositive. *Journal of Health Psychology, 1*, 367-382.

Michal-Johnson, P., & Bowen, S. P. (1992). The place of culture in HIV education. In T. Edgar, M. A. Fitzpatrick, & V. S. Freimuth (Eds.), *AIDS: A communication perspective* (pp. 147-172). Hillsdale, NJ: Lawrence Erlbaum.

Mitchell, M. A. (1989). The relationship between social network variables and the utilization of mental health services. *Journal of Community Psychology, 17*, 258-266.

Monette, P. (1990). *Borrowed time: An AIDS memoir.* New York: Avon.

Monteith, M. J. (1993). Self-regulation of prejudiced responses: Implications for progress in prejudice-reduction efforts. *Journal of Personality and Social Psychology, 65,* 469-485.

Monteith, M. J., Deneen, N. E., & Tooman, G. D. (1996). The effect of social norm activation on the expression of opinions concerning gay men and Blacks. *Basic and Applied Social Psychology, 18,* 267-288.

Moore, J., Solomon, L., Schoenbaum, E., Schuman, P., & Boland, B. (1996, July). *Depressive symptoms and coping strategies among HIV-infected and HIV-uninfected women in four urban centers.* Paper presented at the XI International Conference on AIDS, Vancouver, British Columbia.

Moos, R. H., & Moos, B. S. (1993). *Family environment scale manual* (2nd ed.). Palo Alto, CA: Consulting Psychologists Press.

Morales, E. S. (1983, August). *Third World gays and lesbians: A process of multiple identities.* Paper presented at the 91st Annual Convention of the American Psychological Association, Anaheim, CA.

Moss, A. R., & Bacchetti, P. (1989). Natural history of HIV infection. *AIDS, 3*(2), 55-61.

Moulton, J., Stempel, R., Bacchetti, P., Temoshok, L., & Moos, A. (1991). Results of a one-year longitudinal study of HIV antibody test notification from San Francisco General Hospital cohort. *Journal of Acquired Immune Deficiency Syndrome, 4,* 787-794.

Mullen, B., & Hu, L. T. (1989). Perceptions of ingroup and outgroup variability: A meta-analytic integration. *Basic and Applied Social Psychology, 10,* 233-252.

Namir, S., Alumbaugh, M., Fawzy, F., & Wolcott, D. (1989). The relationship of social support to physical and psychological aspects of AIDS. *Psychology and Health, 3,* 77-86.

Namir, S., Wolcott, D. L., Fawzy, F. L., & Alumbaugh, M. J. (1987). Coping with AIDS: Psychological and health implications. *Journal of Applied Social Psychology, 17,* 309-328.

Nardi, P. M. (1990). AIDS and obituaries: The perpetuation of stigma in the press. In D. A. Feldman (Ed.), *Culture and AIDS* (pp. 159-168). Westport, CT: Praeger.

National Research Council (U.S.) Panel on Monitoring the Social Impact of the AIDS Epidemic. (1993). *The social impact of AIDS in the United States.* Washington, DC: National Academy Press.

Nicholson, W. D., & Long, B. C. (1990). Self-esteem, social support, internalized homophobia, and coping strategies of HIV+ gay men. *Journal of Consulting and Clinical Psychology, 58,* 873-876.

Nisbett, R. E., & Wilson, T. D. (1977). Telling more than we can know: Verbal reports on mental processes. *Psychological Review, 84,* 231-259.

Norton, R., Schwartzbaum, J., & Wheat, J. (1990). Language discrimination of general physicians: AIDS metaphors used in the AIDS crisis. *Communication Research, 17,* 809-826.

O'Brien, K., Wortman, C. B., Kessler, R. C., & Joseph, J. G. (1993). Social relationships of men at risk for AIDS. *Social Science and Medicine, 36,* 1161-1167.

Omoto, A. M. (1989). *Relationship involvement and closeness: Implications for the processing of relationship-relevant events.* Unpublished doctoral dissertation, University of Minnesota, Minneapolis.

Omoto, A. M., & Crain, A. L. (1995a). AIDS volunteerism: Lesbian and gay community-based responses to HIV. In G. M. Herek & B. Greene (Eds.), *Psychological perspectives on lesbian and gay issues: Vol. 2. AIDS, identity, and community: The HIV epidemic and lesbians and gay men* (pp. 187-209). Thousand Oaks, CA: Sage.

Omoto, A. M., & Crain, A. L. (1995b, May). *Stigmatization and volunteerism: Are AIDS volunteers punished for their good deeds?* Paper presented at the meeting of the Midwestern Psychological Association, Chicago, IL.

Omoto, A. M., & Snyder, M. (1990). Basic research in action: Volunteerism and society's response to AIDS. *Personality and Social Psychology Bulletin, 16,* 152-165.

Omoto, A. M., & Snyder, M. (1993). AIDS volunteers and their motivations: Theoretical issues and practical concerns. *Nonprofit Management and Leadership, 4,* 157-176.

Omoto, A. M., & Snyder, M. (1995). Sustained helping without obligation: Motivation, longevity of service, and perceived attitude change among AIDS volunteers. *Journal of Personality and Social Psychology, 68,* 671-686.

Omoto, A. M., Snyder, M., & Berghuis, J. P. (1993). The psychology of volunteerism: A conceptual analysis and a program of action research. In J. B. Pryor & G. D. Reeder (Eds.), *The social psychology of HIV infection* (pp. 333-356). Hillsdale, NJ: Lawrence Erlbaum.

Omoto, A. M., Snyder, M., & Crain, A. L. (1998). *On the stigmatization of people who do good work: The case of AIDS volunteers.* Unpublished manuscript, University of Kansas, Lawrence.

Ostrom, T. M., & Sedikides, C. (1992). Out-group homogeneity effects in natural and minimal groups. *Psychological Bulletin, 112,* 536-552.

Ostrow, D. G., Monjan, A., Joseph, J., VanRaden, M., Fox, R., Kingsley, L., Dudley, J., & Phair, J. (1989). HIV-related symptoms and psychological functioning in a cohort of homosexual men. *American Journal of Psychiatry, 146,* 737-742.

Ouellette, S. C., Cassel, B., Maslanka, H., & Wong, L. M. (1995). GMHC volunteers and the challenges and hopes for the second decade of AIDS. *AIDS Education and Prevention, 7,* 64-79.

Pakenham, K. I., Dadds, M. R., & Terry, D. J. (1994). Relationships between adjustment to HIV and both social support and coping. *Journal of Consulting and Clinical Psychology, 62,* 1194-1203.

Pakenham, K. I., Dadds, M. R., & Terry, D. (1995). Carers' burden and adjustment to HIV. *AIDS Care, 7*(2), 189-203.

Pargament, K. I., Ensing, D. S., Falgout, K., Olsen, H., Reilly, B., Van Haitsma, K., & Warren, R. (1990). God help me: (1): Religious coping efforts as predictors of the outcomes to significant negative life events. *American Journal of Community Psychology, 18,* 793-824.

Parsons, T. (1951). *The social system.* New York: Free Press.

Pearlin, L. I., Mullan, J. T., Aneshensel, C. S., Wardlaw, L., & Harrington, C. (1994). The structure and functions of AIDS caregiving relationships. *Psychosocial Rehabilitation Journal, 17,* 51-67.

Pearson, J. M. (1981). *Talking to terminally ill children about death.* Paper presented at the meeting of the American Academy of Child Psychiatry, Dallas, TX.

Pennebaker, J. W. (1989). Confession, inhibition, and disease. In L. Berkowitz (Ed.), *Advances in experimental social psychology* (Vol. 22, pp. 211-244). New York: Academic Press.

Pennebaker, J. W. (1990). *Opening up: The healing power of confiding in others.* New York: Morrow.

Perry, S., Ryan, J., Fogel, K., Fishman, B., & Jacobsberg, L. (1990). Voluntarily informing others of positive HIV test results: Patterns of notification by infected gay men. *Hospital and Community Psychiatry, 41,* 549-551.

Perry, S. W., Card, C.A.L., Moffatt, M., Ashman, T., Fishman, B., & Jacobsberg, L. B. (1994). Self-disclosure of HIV infection to sexual partners after repeated counseling. *AIDS Education and Prevention, 6,* 403-411.

Peterson, J. L. (1992). Black men and their same-sex desires and behavior. In G. Herdt (Ed.), *Gay culture in America: Essays from the field* (pp. 147-164). Boston, MA: Beacon.

Peterson, J. L. (1995). AIDS-related risks and same-sex behaviors among African American men. In G. M. Herek & B. Greene (Eds.), *Psychological perspectives on lesbian and gay issues: Vol 2. AIDS, identity, and community: The HIV epidemic and lesbians and gay men* (pp. 85-104). Thousand Oaks, CA: Sage.

Peterson, J. L., Coates, T. J., Calaria, J. A., Middleton, L., Hilliard, B., & Hearst, N. (1992). High risk sexual behavior and condom use among gay and bisexual African American men. *American Journal of Public Health, 82,* 1490-1494.

Peterson, J. L., Folkman, S., & Bakeman, R. (1996). Stress, coping, HIV status, psychosocial resources, and depressive mood in African American gay, bisexual, and heterosexual men. *American Journal of Community Psychology, 24,* 461-487.

Peterson, J. L., & Marin, G. (1988). Issues in the prevention of AIDS among Black and Hispanic men. *American Psychologist, 43,* 871-877.

Peterson, Y. (1979). The impact of physical disability on marital adjustment: A literature review. *Family Coordinator, 28,* 47-51.

Petronio, S. (1991). Communication boundary management: A theoretical model of managing disclosure of private information between marital couples. *Communication Theory, 1,* 311-335.

Petronio, S., Martin, J., & Littlefield, R. (1984). Prerequisite conditions for self-disclosure: A gender issue. *Communication Monographs, 51,* 268-273.

Pfuhl, Jr., E. H. (1980). *The deviance process.* New York: Van Nostrand.

Pilisuk, M., & Parks, S. (1986). *The healing web.* Hanover, NH: University Press of New England.

Powell-Cope, G. M., & Brown, M. A. (1992). Going public as an AIDS family caregiver. *Social Science and Medicine, 34,* 571-580.

Prager, K. J. (1995). *The psychology of intimacy.* New York: Guilford.

Pratt, C., Schmall, V., Wright, S., & Cleland, M. (1985). Burden and coping strategies of caregivers to Alzheimer's patients. *Family Relations, 34,* 27-33.

Primomo, J., Yates, B., & Woods, N. (1990). Social support for women during chronic illness: The relationship among sources and types to adjustment. *Research in Nursing Health, 13,* 153-161.

Pryor, J. B., & Reeder, G. D. (1993). Collective and individual representations of HIV/AIDS stigma. In J. B. Pryor & G. D. Reeder (Eds.), *The social psychology of HIV infection* (pp. 263-286). Hillsdale, NJ: Lawrence Erlbaum.

Pryor, J. B., Reeder, G. D., Vinacco, R., & Kot, T. (1989). The instrumental and symbolic functions of attitudes toward people with AIDS. *Journal of Applied Social Psychology, 19,* 377-404.

Quam, M. D. (1990). The sick role, stigma, and pollution: The case of AIDS. In D. A. Feldman (Ed.), *Culture and AIDS* (pp. 29-44). Westport, CT: Praeger.

Query, J. L. Jr., & James, A. C. (1989). The relationship between interpersonal communication competence and social support among elderly support groups in retirement communities. *Journal of Health Communication, 3,* 165-184.

Rabkin, J. G., Williams, J. B., Neugebauer, R., Remien, R. H., & Goetz, R. (1990). Maintenance of hope in HIV-spectrum homosexual men. *American Journal of Psychiatry, 147,* 1322-1326.

Radloff, L. (1977). The CES-D Scale: A self-report depression scale for research in the general population. *Applied Psychological Measurement, 1,* 385-401.

Raveis, V. H., & Siegel, K. (1991, February). The impact of care giving on informal or familial care givers. *AIDS Patient Care,* pp. 39-43.

Reed, P. (1987). Spirituality and well-being in terminally ill hospitalized adults. *Research in Nursing and Health, 10,* 335-344.

Rehm, L. P. (1977). Self-control model of depression. *Behavior Therapy, 8,* 787-804.

Remien, R. H., Rabkin, J. G., Williams, J. B., & Katoff, L. (1992). Coping strategies and health beliefs of AIDS longterm survivors. *Psychology and Health, 6,* 335-345.

Revenson, T. (1994). Social support and marital coping with chronic illness. *Annals of Behavioral Medicine, 16*(2), 122-130.

Revenson, T., & Felton, B. J. (1989). Disability and coping as predictors of psychological adjustment to rheumatoid arthritis. *Journal of Clinical and Consulting Psychology, 57,* 344-348.

Rogers, J. W., & Buffalo, M. D. (1974). Fighting back: Nine modes of adaptation to a deviant label. *Social Problems, 22,* 101-118.

Rolland, J. (1994). In sickness and in health: The impact of illness on couples' relationships. *Journal of Marital and Family Therapy, 20,* 327-347.

Rook, K. S. (1984). The negative side of social interaction: Impact on psychological well-being. *Journal of Personality and Social Psychology, 46,* 1097-1108.

Rosenberg, P. S. (1995). Scope of the AIDS epidemic in the United States. *Science, 270,* 1372-1375.

Rosenberg, P. S., Biggar, R., & Goedert, J. (1994). Declining age at HIV infection in the United States. *New England Journal of Medicine, 330,* 789.

Rosenstock, I. M., & Kirscht, J. (1979). Why people use health services. In A. Stone, F. Cohen, & N. E. Adler (Eds.), *Health psychology* (pp. 189-206). San Francisco, CA: Jossey-Bass.

Samuel, M. C., & Osmond, D. E. (1996). Annotation: Uncertainties in the estimation of HIV prevalence and incidence in the United States. *American Journal of Public Health, 86,* 627-628.

Sarason, I., Sarason, B., Shearin, E., & Pierce, G. (1987). A brief measure of social support: Practical and theoretical implications. *Journal of Social and Personal Relationships, 4,* 497-510.

Savin-Williams, R. C. (1996). Ethnic- and sexual-minority youth. In R. C. Savin-Williams & K. M. Cohen (Eds.), *The lives of lesbians, gays, and bisexuals* (pp. 152-165). Fort Worth, TX: Harcourt, Brace.

Schachter, S. (1951). Deviation, rejection, and communication. *Journal of Abnormal and Social Psychology, 46,* 190-207.

Schachter, S. (1959). *The psychology of affiliation.* Palo Alto, CA: Stanford University Press.

Schaefer, M. T., & Olson, D. H. (1981). Assessing intimacy: The Pair Inventory. *Journal of Marital and Family Therapy, 7,* 640-653.

Schaefer, S., & Coleman, E. (1992). Shifts in meaning, purpose, and values following a diagnosis of human immunodeficiency virus (HIV) infection among gay men. *Journal of Psychology and Human Sexuality, 5,* 13-29.

Schneider, S. G., Taylor, S. E., Hammen, C., Kemeny, M. E., & Dudley, J. (1991). Factors influencing suicide intent in gay and bisexual suicide ideators: Differing models for men with and without human immunodeficiency virus. *Journal of Personality and Social Psychology, 61,* 776-788.

Schnell, D. J., Higgins, D. L., Wilson, R. M., Goldbaum, G., Cohn, D. L., & Wolitski, R. J. (1992). Men's disclosure of HIV test results to male primary sex partners. *American Journal of Public Health, 82,* 1675-1676.

Schulz, R., Tompkins, C., Wood, D., & Deekers, S. C. (1987). The social psychology of care giving: Physical and psychological costs of providing support to the disabled. *Journal of Applied Social Psychology, 17,* 401-428.

Schwartzberg, S. S. (1993). Struggling for meaning: How HIV-positive gay men make sense of AIDS. *Professional Psychology: Research and Practice, 24*(4), 483-490.

Schwarzer, R., Dunkel-Schetter, C., & Kemeny, M. (1994). The multidimensional nature of received social support in gay men at risk of HIV infection and AIDS. *American Journal of Community Psychology, 22,* 319-339.

Schwarzer, R., & Leppin, A. (1989). Social support and health: A meta-analysis. *Psychology and Health: An International Journal, 3,* 1-15.

Schwarzer, R., & Leppin, A. (1991). Social support and health: A theoretical and empirical overview. *Journal of Social and Personal Relationships, 8,* 99-127.

Semple, S., Patterson, T., Temoshok, L., McCutchan, J., Straits-Troster, K., Chandler, J., & Grant, I. (1993). Identification of psychobiological stressors among HIV-positive women. *Women and Health, 20*(4), 15-36.

Serovich, J. M., & Greene, K. (1993). Perceptions of family boundaries: The case of disclosure of HIV testing information. *Family Relations, 42,* 193-197.

Serovich, J. M., Greene, K., & Parrott, R. (1992). Boundaries and AIDS testing: Privacy and the family system. *Family Relations, 41,* 104-109.

Serovich, J. M., Kimberly, J. A., & Greene, K. (1998). Perceived family member reaction to women's disclosure of HIV-positive information. *Family Relations, 47,* 15-22.

Shaver, K. G. (1970). Defensive attribution: Effects of severity and relevance on the responsibility assigned for an accident. *Journal of Personality and Social Psychology, 14,* 101-113.

Shelp, E. E., DuBose, E. R., & Sunderland, R. H. (1990). The infrastructure of religious communities: A neglected resource for care of people with AIDS. *American Journal of Public Health, 80,* 970-972.

Shilts, R. (1987). *And the band played on: Politics, people, and the AIDS epidemic.* New York: St. Martin's Press.

Shrauger, J. S., & Schoeneman, T. J. (1979). Symbolic interactionist view of self-concept: Through the looking glass darkly. *Psychological Bulletin, 86,* 549-573.

Siegel, K., & Krauss, B. J. (1991). Living with HIV infection: Adaptive tasks of seropositive gay men. *Journal of Health and Social Behavior, 32,* 17-32.

Sigelman, C. K., Howell, J. L., Cornell, D. P., Cutright, J. D., & Dewey, J. C. (1991). Courtesy stigma: The social implications of associating with a gay person. *Journal of Social Psychology, 131,* 45-56.

Silver, R. L., Boon, C., & Stones, M. H. (1983). Searching for meaning in misfortune: Making sense of incest. *Journal of Social Issues, 39,* 81-102.

Simoni, J. M., Mason, H.R.C., Marks, G., Ruiz, M. S., Reed, D., & Richardson, J. L. (1995). Women's self-disclosure of HIV infection: Rates, reasons, and reactions. *Journal of Consulting and Clinical Psychology, 63,* 474-478.

Smith, D. K., & Moore, J. (1996). Epidemiology, manifestations, and treatment of HIV infection in women. In A. O'Leary & L. S. Jemmott (Eds.), *Women and AIDS: Coping and Care* (pp. 1-32). New York: Plenum.

Snyder, M., & Omoto, A. M. (1992). Volunteerism and society's response to the HIV epidemic. *Current Directions in Psychological Science, 1,* 113-115.

Snyder, M., Omoto, A. M., & Crain, A. L. (1997). *Punished for their good deeds: Stigmatization of AIDS volunteers*. Manuscript submitted for pubication.

Snyder, M., Omoto, A. M., & Crain, A. L. (1996b, April). *Punished for their good deeds: The stigmatization of AIDS volunteers*. Paper presented at the National Institute of Mental Health workshop on AIDS and stigma research, Rockville, MD.

Sontag, S. (1979). *Illness as metaphor*. New York: Vintage.

Spiegel, D., Bloom, J. R., Kraemer, H. C., & Gottheil, E. (1989, October 14). Effect of psychosocial treatment on survival of patients with metastatic breast cancer. *Lancet*, 888-891.

Steele, T. E., Finkelstein, S. H., & Finkelstein, F. O. (1976). Marital discord, sexual problems, and depression. *Journal of Nervous and Mental Disorders, 162*, 225-237.

Stempel, R. R., Moulton, J. M., & Moss, A. R. (1995). Self-disclosure of HIV-1 antibody test results: The San Francisco General Hospital cohort. *AIDS Education and Prevention, 7*, 116-123.

Stevens, J. (1992). *Applied multivariate statistics for the social sciences* (2nd ed.). Hillsdale, NJ: Lawrence Erlbaum.

St. Lawrence, J. S., Husfeldt, B. A., Kelly, J. A., Hood, H. V., & Smith, S. (1990). The stigma of AIDS: Fear of disease and prejudice toward gay men. *Journal of Homosexuality, 19*, 85-101.

Stokes, J. P., McKirnan, D. J., & Burzette, R. G. (1993). Sexual behavior, condom use, disclosure of sexuality, and stability of sexual orientation in bisexual men. *Journal of Sex Research, 30*, 203-213.

Stulberg, I., & Buchingham, S. L. (1988, June). Parallel issues for AIDS patients, families, and others. *Social Casework: The Journal of Contemporary Social Work*, 355-359.

Sullivan, A. (1996, November 10). When plague ends: Notes on the twilight of an epidemic. *New York Times Magazine*, pp. 52-58, 60-62, 76-78.

Suls, J., & Fletcher, B. (1985). The relative efficacy of avoidant and non-avoidant coping strategies: A meta-analysis. *Health Psychology, 4*, 249-288.

Susman, J. R. (1988). Disclosure of traumas and psychosomatic processes. *Social Science and Medicine, 26*, 327-332.

Tajfel, H., & Turner, J. C. (1986). The social identity theory of intergroup behavior. In S. Worchel & W. G. Austin (Eds.), *Psychology of intergroup relations* (pp. 2-24). Chicago: Nelson-Hall.

Tasker, M. (1992). *How can I tell you?* Bethesda, MD: Association for the Care of Children's Health.

Taylor, S. E. (1983). Adjustment to threatening events: A theory of cognitive adaptation. *American Psychologist, 38*, 1161-1173.

Taylor, S. E., & Dakof, G. A. (1987). Social support and the cancer patient. In S. Spacapan & S. Oskamp (Eds.), *The social psychology of health* (pp. 95-116). Newbury Park, CA: Sage.

Taylor, S. E., Falke, R. L., Mazel, R. M., Hilsberg, B. L. (1988). Sources of satisfaction and dissatisfaction among members of cancer support groups. In B. H. Gottlieb (Ed.), *Marshaling social support: Formats, processes, and effects* (pp. 187-208). Newbury Park, CA: Sage.

Taylor, S. E., Lichtman, R. R., & Wood, J. V. (1984). Attributions, beliefs about control and adjustment to breast cancer. *Journal of Personality and Social Psychology, 46*, 489-502.

Teguis, A. (1992). Dying with AIDS. In P. I. Ahmed & N. Ahmed (Ed.), *Living and dying with AIDS* (pp. 153-177). New York: Plenum.

Terr, L. (1983). Chowchilla revisited: The effects of psychic trauma four years after a school bus kidnapping. *American Journal of Psychiatry, 140*, 1543-1550.

Thibaut, J. W., & Kelley, H. H. (1958). *The social psychology of groups.* New York: Wiley.

Tremble, B., Schneider, M., & Appathurai, C. (1989). Growing up gay or lesbian in a multicultural context. *Journal of Homosexuality, 17*(3-4), 253-267.

Trobst, K., Collins, R., & Embree, J. (1994). The role of emotion in social support provision: Gender empathy and expression of distress. *Journal of Social and Personal Relationships, 11,* 45-62.

Turner, H. A., Catania, J. A., & Gagnon, J. (1994). The prevalence of informal caregiving to persons with AIDS in the United States: Caregiver characteristics and their implications. *Social Science Medicine, 38,* 1543-1552.

van den Borne, H. W., Pruyn, J. F. A., & van den Heuvel, W. J. A. (1987). Effects of contacts between cancer patients on their psychosocial problems. *Patient Education and Counseling, 9,* 33-51.

van Yperen, N. W., Buunk, B. P., & Schaufeli, W. B. (1992). Communal orientation and the burnout syndrome among nurses. *Journal of Applied Social Psychology, 22,* 173-189.

Velentgas, P., Bynum, C., & Zierler, S. (1990). The buddy volunteer commitment in AIDS care. *American Journal of Public Health, 80,* 1378-1380.

Vitaliano, P., Katon, W., Maiuro, R. D., & Russo, J. (1989). Coping in chest pain patients with and without psychiatric disorders. *Journal of Consulting and Clinical Psychology, 57,* 338-343.

Walster, E. (1966). Assignment of responsibility for an accident. *Journal of Personality and Social Psychology, 3,* 73-79.

Walster, E., Walster, G. W., & Berscheid, E. (1978). *Equity: Theory and research.* Rockleigh, NJ: Allyn and Bacon.

Watney, S. (1986). Common knowledge. *High Performance, 36,* 44-47.

Watney, S. (1987). *Policing desire: Pornography, AIDS, and the media.* Minneapolis: University of Minnesota Press.

Weiner, B., Perry, R. P., & Magnusson, J. (1988). An attributional analysis of reactions to stigmas. *Journal of Personality and Social Psychology, 55,* 738-748.

Weitz, R. (1990). Living with the stigma of AIDS. *Qualitative Sociology, 13,* 23-38.

Wellisch, D., Jamison, R., & Pasnau, R. (1978). Psychological aspects of mastectomy. II. The man's perspective. *American Journal of Psychiatry, 135,* 543-545.

Westbrook, M. T., & Viney, L. I. (1983). Age and sex differences in patients' reactions to illness. *Journal of Health and Social Behavior, 24,* 313-324.

Wiener, L. S., & Septimus, A. (1994). Psychosocial support for the child and family. In P. A. Pizzo & C. M. Wilfert (Eds.), *Pediatric AIDS* (2nd ed., pp. 809-828). Baltimore: Williams & Wilkins.

Williams, M. J. (1988). Gay men as buddies to persons living with AIDS and ARC. *Smith College Studies in Social Work, 59,* 38-52.

Wills, T. A. (1990). Multiple networks and substance use. *Journal of Social and Clinical Psychology, 9,* 78-90.

Wolcott, D. L., Namir, S. N., Fawzy, F. I., Gottlieb, M. S., & Mistuyasu, R. T. (1986). Illness concerns, attitudes towards homosexuality, and social support in gay men with AIDS. *General Hospital Psychiatry, 8,* 395-403.

Wolf, T. M., Balson, P. M., Morse, E. V., Simon, P. M., Gaumer, R. H., Dralle, P. W., & Williams, M. H. (1991). Relationship of coping style to affective state and perceived social support in asymptomatic and symptomatic HIV-infected persons: Implications for clinical management. *Journal of Clinical Psychiatry, 52,* 171-173.

Wood, J. V., Taylor, S. E., & Lichtman, R. R. (1985). Social comparison in adjustment to breast cancer. *Journal of Personality and Social Psychology, 49,* 1169-1183.

Woods, N., Haberman, M., & Packard, N. (1993). Demands of illness and individual, dyadic, and family adaptation in chronic illness. *Western Journal of Nursing Research,*
15(1), 10-30.

World Health Organization Global AIDS Statistics. (1997). *Aids Care, 9,* 251-255.

Worth, D. (1990). Minority women and AIDS: Culture, race and gender. In D. A. Feldman
(Ed.), *Culture and AIDS* (pp. 111-135). New York: Praeger.

Wright, L. (1991). The impact of Alzheimer's disease on the marital relationship. *The*
Gerontologist, 31, 224-237.

Yalom, I. D. (1980). *Existential psychotherapy.* New York: Basic Books.

Yalom, I. D. (1985). *The theory and practice of group psychotherapy* (3rd ed.). New York:
Basic Books.

Yankeelov, P. A. (1995). *The process of departure navigation.* Unpublished doctoral dissertation, University of Louisville.

Yep, G. A. (1993, November). *Disclosure of HIV infection to significant others: A commu-*
nication boundary management perspective. Paper presented at the meeting of the
Speech Communication Association, Miami, FL.

Zich, J., & Temoshok, L. (1987). Perceptions of social support in men with AIDS and ARC:
Relationships with distress and hardiness. *Journal of Applied Social Psychology, 17,*
193-215.

Index

Avoidance, 44. *See also* Avoidance
behaviors; Avoidant coping strategies
Avoidance behaviors, 88, 92, 95
Avoidant coping strategies, 49, 180-181,
189-190, 226, 229-330

Barbee, Anita P., x, 1, 11, 83, 84, 86, 87,
90, 93, 95, 102, 147n, 220, 222,
227, 228
Barbee Interactive Coping Behavior
Coding System (ICBCS), 90
Battles, Haven B., 193
Beck, A. T., 217n
Beck Depression Inventory, 202-203
Behavior:
approach, 87, 92, 95
at-risk, 5
avoidance, 88, 92, 95. *See also*
Avoidance behaviors
dismiss, 87, 90, 92, 94
escape, 88, 90, 92, 94-95
solace, 87, 90, 92-96, 101
solve, 87, 90, 93, 95-96, 101
Behavioral avoidance, 44
Bereavement, 38, 61, 72. *See also*
Mourning
Berghuis, J., 180
Black community, 59, 75
Black gay men:
seropositive, 56-82
similarities to White gay men, 65-72
sociocultural context of AIDS for,
58-63
Blacks. *See* African Americans;
Black community; Black gay men
Blacks Assisting Blacks Against AIDS
(BABAA), 56n, 64, 67, 80
Blame, 41-42, 50-54
Blood transfusion, 17, 99
Bonaventure House, 137-146
Boundry management, theory of, 224
Bowen, S. P., 236
Braithwaite, D. O., 197
Bronchitis, 67
Brown, M. A., 214-215

Catharsis, 153, 161
Cawyer, C. S., 133, 134
Center for Epidemiologic Studies
Depression Scale (CES-D), 183

Centers for Disease Control and
Prevention (CDC), 3, 168, 193-194
Chauncey, S., 85
Children:
HIV-infected, 193-217
of HIV-infected women, 231
number of AIDS cases in, 193
sexually abused, 61
virus transfer to, 5
Church:
in Black community, 62
needs of PWAs and, 130
See also Religion; Spirituality
Clergy, support from, 91
Closeness:
self-disclosure and, 153
of volunteer-PWA relationship, 116-128
Cognitive avoidance, 44
Cognitive readjustment process, 57
Coleman, E., 63, 64, 65, 73, 74, 77, 78,
79, 80, 81
Collins, Rebecca L., 11, 30, 40, 45, 51,
52, 53, 231
Communication, 168, 174-175
Community HIV/AIDS organizations,
234-235
Concealment, 24, 61, 147-163. *See also*
Nondisclosure; Passing
Coopersmith, S., 197
Coping:
active, 84, 180, 229-330
avoidant, 49, 180-181, 189-190, 226.
See also Avoidance; Avoidance
behaviors; Avoidant coping
strategies
Black gay men, 56, 68-70
depression and, 190-191
disclosure and, 163
gay social identity and, 30-55
HIV-serodiscordant heterosexual
couples, 178-179
interactive, 103-104
interpersonal, 10
intimacy and, 181
personal, 10
positive, 136
problem-solving, 226
relationships and, 182, 185, 226
self-identity and, 10
self-presentational, 45

stigma and, 233
Homosexuality:
Blacks and, 75, 79-80. *See also* Black
gay men
concealment of Black gay men's, 61
disclosure of, 149
ethnic minorities' denial of, 59
homosexuals' attitudes toward, 52
negative attitudes toward, 49, 51
Reagan adminsitration and, 25
stigma on, 31
Honesty, 153-154
Hostility, 23
Human immunodeficiency virus (HIV).
See HIV

ICBCS. *See* Barbee Interactive Coping
Behavior Coding System
Identity, 228
Incidence, 5
Informal caregivers, 130. *See also* AIDS
volunteers
Informal support, 132, 135-137, 141-142
Informational support, 135
Injection drug use, 58, 61, 169.
See also Intravenous drug use
Internalized homophobia, 43
International Conference on AIDS (XI),
219
Interpersonal disassociation, 14-21
Interpersonal relationships, 21-23, 135-137
Intimacy:
coping and, 181, 185, 190
in HIV-serodiscordant heterosexual
couples, 168, 174
Intravenous drug use, 3, 17, 99, 137, 177.
See also Injection drug use
Invasion, 134

Jacobsberg, L., 149
Job status, 97. *See also* Employment
Johnson, Magic, 23
Jones, E. E., 14
Jones, Johnny, 70, 78

Kaposi's sarcoma, 19, 26
Kelly, J. J., 85
Kennedy, Cheryl A., 165
Kimberly, J. A., 223

Klein, K., 180

Lackner, J. B., 49
Leary, Mark R., 11, 12, 16, 19, 24, 196,
230, 234
Lehman, D. R., 95
Lesbian, 236
Leserman, J., 85, 136
Lesondak, Linda M., 165
Levin, B. W., 195
Libow, J., 198-199
Limandri, B. J., 195-196
Long, B. C., 49
Loss, 134
Lovejoy, David, 11, 147
Lover, 91-92, 103. *See also* Relationship
partner; Sexual partner
Loyalty, 153, 161

Magnusson, J., 194
Manne, S. L., 180
Mark of deviance, 14
Marks, G., 149, 225
Mason, H. R. C., 149
Meaning:
defensive, 67-70
high, 66-68
of HIV, 65-72
irrelevant, 69-72
search for, 57. *See also* Search for
meaning
shattered, 69-71
specific sources of, 73-80
Media, 198, 207
Mediating structures, 131-135, 142
Michal-Johnson, P., 236
Minorities:
homophobia among ethnic, 59
incidence of HIV/AIDS among, 5
Mitsuyasu, R. T., 49
Monahan, J. L., 237
Monteith, M. J., 54-55, 235
Moore, Jan, 11, 165, 166, 171
Moralizing, 130
Mother, 84
Mourning, 130. *See also* Bereavement

Namir, S. N., 49
Nardi, P. M., 22-23

About the Editors

Valerian J. Derlega, PhD, is Professor of Psychology at Old Dominion University, Norfolk, Virginia. He received his doctoral degree in social psychology from the University of Maryland in 1971. His research interests include self-disclosure and privacy regulation in close relationships, social support and coping with stress, the impact of the male role on relationships, and therapy as a personal relationship. He recently coauthored two books, *Self-Disclosure* and *Gender and Close Relationships*.

Anita P. Barbee, PhD, is Associate Research Professor in the Kent School of Social Work at the University of Louisville in Kentucky. She received her doctoral degree in social psychology from the University of Georgia in 1988. She was recently given the 1997 G. R. Miller Early Career Award by the International Network on Personal Relationships for her experimental studies on interactive coping in close relationships. She has published in various journals such as *Journal of Personality and Social Psychology* and *Communication Yearbook* on helping, social support, and relationship formation and is on the editorial boards of the *Journal of Social and Personal Relationships* and *Motivation and Emotion*.